Basic Science Insights into Clinical Puzzles

Editor

JOHN J. DIGIOVANNA

DERMATOLOGIC CLINICS

www.derm.theclinics.com

Consulting Editor
BRUCE H. THIERS

January 2017 • Volume 35 • Number 1

ELSEVIER

1600 John F. Kennedy Boulevard • Suite 1800 • Philadelphia, Pennsylvania, 19103-2899

http://www.theclinics.com

DERMATOLOGIC CLINICS Volume 35, Number 1
January 2017 ISSN 0733-8635, ISBN-13: 978-0-323-48259-2

Editor: Jessica McCool
Developmental Editor: Alison Swety

Dermatologic Clinics (ISSN 0733-8635) is published quarterly by Elsevier Inc., 360 Park Avenue South, New York, NY 10010-1710. Months of publication are January, April, July, and October. Business and editorial offices: 1600 John F. Kennedy Blvd., Suite 1800, Philadelphia, PA 19103-2899. Customer service office: 11830 Westline Drive, St. Louis, MO 63146. Periodicals postage paid at New York, NY, and additional mailing offices. Subscription prices are USD 377.00 per year for US individuals, USD 655.00 per year for US institutions, USD 434.00 per year for Canadian individuals, USD 799.00 per year for Canadian institutions, USD 505.00 per year for international individuals, USD 799.00 per year for international institutions, USD 100.00 per year for US students/residents, and USD 240.00 per year for Canadian and international students/residents. International air speed delivery is included in all *Clinics* subscription prices. All prices are subject to change without notice. **POSTMASTER:** Send address changes to *Dermatologic Clinics*, Elsevier Health Sciences Division, Subscription Customer Service, 3251 Riverport Lane, Maryland Heights, MO 63043. **Customer Service: 1-800-654-2452 (U.S. and Canada); 314-447-8871 (outside U.S. and Canada). Fax: 314-447-8029. E-mail: journalscustomerservice-usa@elsevier.com (for print support); journalsonlinesupport-usa@elsevier.com (for online support).**

Reprints. For copies of 100 or more, of articles in this publication, please contact the Commercial Reprints Department, Elsevier Inc., 360 Park Avenue South, New York, New York 10010-1710. Tel.: 212-633-3874; Fax: 212-633-3820; Email: reprints@elsevier.com.

The *Dermatologic Clinics* is covered in *MEDLINE/PubMed (Index Medicus)*, *Current Contents/Clinical Medicine*, *Excerpta Medica*, *Chemical Abstracts,* and *ISI/BIOMED*.

Contributors

CONSULTING EDITOR

BRUCE H. THIERS, MD
Professor and Chairman, Department of
Dermatology and Dermatologic Surgery,
Medical University of South Carolina,
Charleston, South Carolina

EDITOR

JOHN J. DiGIOVANNA, MD
Senior Research Physician, DNA Repair
Section, Dermatology Branch, Center for
Cancer Research, National Cancer Institute,
Bethesda, Maryland

AUTHORS

LESLIE G. BIESECKER, MD
Chief and Senior Investigator, Medical
Genomics and Metabolic Genetics Branch,
National Human Genome Research Institute,
National Institutes of Health, Bethesda,
Maryland

JOHN A. CARUCCI, MD, PhD
The Ronald O. Perelman Department of
Dermatology, New York University School of
Medicine, New York, New York

IJEURU CHIKEKA, MD
Department of Biochemistry and Molecular
Biology, University of Maryland School of
Medicine, Baltimore, Maryland

THOMAS N. DARLING, MD, PhD
Professor and Chair, Department of
Dermatology, Uniformed Services University of
the Health Sciences, Bethesda, Maryland

DIMANA DIMITROVA, MD
Clinical Fellow, Experimental Transplantation
and Immunology Branch, National Cancer
Institute, National Institutes of Health,
Bethesda, Maryland

ANNA DUBOIS, BSc, MBChB
Department of Dermatology, Royal Victoria
Infirmary, Newcastle upon Tyne, United
Kingdom

DIANE FELSEN, PhD
Department of Urology, Institute for Pediatric
Urology, Weill Cornell Medical College,
New York, New York

ALEXANDRA F. FREEMAN, MD
Staff Clinician, Laboratory of Clinical Infectious
Diseases, National Institute of Allergy and
Infectious Diseases, National Institutes of
Health, Bethesda, Maryland

RICHARD L. GALLO, MD, PhD
Professor and Chair, Department of
Dermatology, University of California, San
Diego, San Diego, California

**RAPHAELA GOLDBACH-MANSKY, MD,
MHS**
Investigator, Head, Translational
Autoinflammatory Disease Studies, National
Institute of Allergy and Infectious Diseases,
National Institutes of Health, Bethesda,
Maryland

KIRSTY HODGSON, BSc, MRes
Institute of Genetic Medicine, Newcastle
University, Newcastle upon Tyne, United
Kingdom

THOMAS J. HORNYAK, MD, PhD
Associate Professor, Department of
Biochemistry and Molecular Biology,
University of Maryland School of Medicine,
Research & Development Service, VA
Maryland Health Care System, Associate
Professor, Department of Dermatology,
University of Maryland School of Medicine,
Baltimore, Maryland

JENNIFER M. HUANG, PhD
Department of Biochemistry and Molecular
Biology, University of Maryland School of
Medicine, Baltimore, Maryland

KIM M. KEPPLER-NOREUIL, MD
Senior Staff Clinician, Medical Genomics and
Metabolic Genetics Branch, National Human
Genome Research Institute, National Institutes
of Health, Bethesda, Maryland

CHYI-CHIA RICHARD LEE, MD, PhD
Staff Clinician, Dermatopathology Section,
Laboratory of Pathology, Center for Cancer
Research, National Cancer Institute, National
Institutes of Health, Bethesda, Maryland

JOEL MOSS, MD, PhD
Deputy Chief and Senior Investigator,
Cardiovascular and Pulmonary Branch,
National Heart, Lung, and Blood Institute,
National Institutes of Health, Bethesda,
Maryland

NEERA NATHAN, MD
Department of Dermatology, Uniformed
Services University of the Health Sciences,
Bethesda, Maryland

NEIL RAJAN, MBBS, PhD
Institute of Genetic Medicine, Newcastle
University, Department of Dermatology, Royal
Victoria Infirmary, Newcastle upon Tyne,
United Kingdom

ALEXIS L. SANTANA, PhD
The Ronald O. Perelman Department of
Dermatology, New York University School of
Medicine, New York, New York

TIFFANY C. SCHARSCHMIDT, MD
Assistant Professor, Department of
Dermatology, University of California, San
Francisco, San Francisco, California

KYAWT WIN SHWIN, MD
Associate Professor, Division of Rheumatic
Diseases, UT Southwestern Medical Center,
Dallas VA Medical Center, North Texas Health
Care System, Dallas, Texas; Translational
Autoinflammatory Disease Studies,
Rheumatology Fellowship Program, National
Institutes of Arthritis and Musculoskeletal and
Skin Diseases, National Institutes of Health,
Bethesda, Maryland

TOSHIYA TAKAHASHI, MD, PhD
Postdoctoral Fellow, Department of
Dermatology, University of California, San
Diego, San Diego, California

DAVID T. WOODLEY, MD
Professor, Emeritus Founding Chair,
Department of Dermatology, The Keck School
of Medicine, University of Southern California,
Los Angeles, California

Contents

Antimicrobials, Immunity, and Inflammation: When to Do Battle, and How

Commensal bacteria live intimately and in constant dialogue with skin immune cells. Regulating our immune response to these bacteria is critical for skin homeostasis. Using a new murine model to track *Staphylococcus epidermidis*-specific T cells, we found that colonization during neonatal but not adult life led to *S.epidermidis*-specific immune tolerance. This tolerance protected against skin inflammation and was mediated by a wave of regulatory T cells entering neonatal skin. These findings provide new insight into how we establish a healthy symbiosis with commensal microbes and highlight avenues for future research to identify novel therapies for inflammatory skin disease.

DOCK8 deficiency is an autosomal recessive combined immunodeficiency disease associated with elevated IgE, atopy, recurrent sinopulmonary and cutaneous viral infections, and malignancy. The DOCK8 protein is critical for cytoskeletal organization, and deficiency impairs dendritic cell transmigration, T-cell survival, and NK cell cytotoxicity. Early hematopoietic stem cell transplantation is gaining prominence as a definitive treatment given the potential for severe complications and mortality in this disease. Recently, DOCK2 deficiency has been identified in several patients with early-onset invasive bacterial and viral infections.

Autoinflammatory disorders are sterile inflammatory conditions characterized by episodes of early-onset fever, rash, and disease-specific patterns of organ inflammation. Gain-of-function mutations in innate danger-sensing pathways, including the inflammasomes and the nucleic acid sensing pathways, play critical roles in the pathogenesis of IL-1 and Type-I IFN-mediated disorders and point to an important role of excessive proinflammatory cytokine signaling, including interleukin (IL)-1b , Type-I interferons, IL-18, TNF and others in causing the organ specific immune dysregulation. The article discusses the concept of targeting proinflammatory cytokines and their signaling pathways with cytokine blocking treatments that have been life changing for some patients.

Genetics, Lineage, and Malignancy

Infrequently, melanocytic nevi undergo malignant transformation to melanoma. Understanding molecular and cellular mechanisms underlying oncogene-induced senescence should help identify pathways underlying melanoma development, leading to the development of new strategies for melanoma prevention and early detection.

Human skin wounds heal largely by reparative wound healing rather than regenerative wound healing. Human skin wounds heal with scarring and without pilosebaceous units or other appendages. Dermal fibroblasts come from 2 distinct lineages of cells that have distinct cell markers and, more importantly, distinct functional abilities. Human skin wound healing largely involves the dermal fibroblast lineage from the reticular dermis and not the papillary dermis. If scientists could find a way to stimulate the dermal fibroblast lineages from the papillary dermis in early wound healing, perhaps human skin wounds could heal without scarring and with skin appendages.

DERMATOLOGIC CLINICS

THE CLINICS ARE AVAILABLE ONLINE!
Access your subscription at:
www.theclinics.com

Preface
Basic Science Insights into Clinical Puzzles

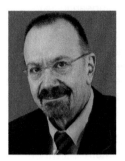

John J. DiGiovanna, MD

Editor

Dermatologists are curious, perhaps because what we see in clinic often challenges our understanding. Several recent scientific advances have yielded breakthroughs that help explain some clinical mysteries. I've asked these cutting-edge, basic and translational scientists to summarize their recent work that has helped answer some of the puzzling questions that arise in the clinic.

"So THAT'S how that happens!"

From birth, maybe even earlier, we learn how to interact with our environment. Our immune systems react fiercely to organisms like *Staphylococcus aureus*, yet develop tolerance to commensals like *Staphylococcus epidermidis*. Tiffany Scharschmidt (University of California, San Francisco) has uncovered some of the secrets of how and when our immune systems define friend versus foe, and the multiple dimensions involved.

Most warts resolve, sometimes spontaneously, while others do not. Why is one family member severely affected? Is it the difference in the virus, host, or some other factor? Drs Dimitrova and Freeman (NIH) describe the recently identified inherited disorders of DOCK8 and DOCK2 deficiency, which help understand why some patients develop widespread, recalcitrant disease, and how the dermatologist can be key to the early diagnosis of these disorders.

A series of autoinflammatory disorders with profound dermatologic manifestations have recently been characterized, not only clinically but also with a detailed understanding of underlying genetic mutations and inflammatory pathways. This has led to some highly effective, specific therapies. Raphaela Goldbach-Mansky and her team (NIH) have been instrumental in leading this discovery. They show us how to identify these disorders and understand their diverse skin presentations.

Why doesn't psoriatic skin become infected, even after surgery, compared with other inflammatory skin conditions, like eczema? Why is atopic dermatitis skin prone to colonization and infection with *S aureus*? Why is rosacea flared by sun—could it be related to vitamin D? Richard Gallo and his team (University of California, San Diego) have led the discovery of antimicrobial peptides in skin and their relationship to a spectrum of diseases.

Early on, I was taught that every somatic cell in my body had identical genetic makeup. With the understanding that premalignant cells, such as keratinocytes, harbor DNA damage, it became clear that genetic mosaicism is widespread. Each of us is a mosaic. Depending on when in development the mosaicism occurs and which cell lineages are involved results in varied clinical presentation. Certain disorders can help us understand mosaicism, just as understanding mosaicism can help us understand disease pathogenesis. Tom Darling's team (Uniformed Services University and NIH) studies somatic mutations in the mTORC1 signaling pathway, and they explain how mosaicism affects clinical presentation and implications for therapy.

Dermatol Clin 35 (2017) ix–x
http://dx.doi.org/10.1016/j.det.2016.10.001
0733-8635/17/© 2016 Published by Elsevier Inc.

derm.theclinics.com

While cylindromas were described over 150 years ago, it was the discovery of underlying *CYLD* mutations that demonstrated the link between several clinical syndromes. Neil Rajan and his team (Newcastle University, UK) describe this relationship and how understanding the pathophysiology is paving the way toward novel medical interventions for these disfiguring tumors.

Posttransplantation skin cancer is a major cause of morbidity and mortality. Why do patients fare worse on cyclosporine compared with other agents, such as sirolimus. John Carucci and his team (NYU) dissect the complex relationship between cyclosporine and interleukin-22 to uncover the interaction between the immune system, immunosuppression, and skin cancer and suggest new avenues to explore to harness this difficult management problem.

Approximately half of melanomas carry a mutation in the gene that encodes BRAF, a proto-oncogene involved in sending growth signals from outside cells to the nucleus. It is part of the RAS/MAPK pathway. Vemurafenib and dabrafenib, which target the BRAF V600E mutation, have been approved for metastatic melanoma. It is puzzling then, why this melanoma-associated mutation should be commonly present in benign nevi. Tom Hornyak's research team (University of Maryland/Baltimore VA) describes how oncogene-induced senescence may explain the paradox.

The physical, cosmetic, financial, and psychological burden from scars induced by burns, trauma, surgery, and combat is daunting. Re-creating a more normal-appearing skin, with reticular and papillary dermis housing adnexal structures like hair follicles and sweat glands, could mitigate this morbidity. David Woodley (UCLA) describes newly identified features of fibroblasts that distinguish between different types of dermis, suggesting the first steps in the pathway from amorphous scar to regeneration of normal-appearing skin.

I hope you enjoy how these researchers are answering our clinical questions.

John J. DiGiovanna, MD
DNA Repair Section
Dermatology Branch
Center for Cancer Research
National Cancer Institute
NIH, Building 37 Room 4002
Bethesda, MD 20892-4262, USA

E-mail address:
jdg@nih.gov

Establishing Tolerance to Commensal Skin Bacteria
Timing Is Everything

Tiffany C. Scharschmidt, MD

KEYWORDS

- Skin • Microbiome • Tregs • Tolerance • Neonatal • Commensals

KEY POINTS

- Our skin is home to many commensal bacteria that normally do not cause disease.
- Regulating our immune response, that is, establishing tolerance, to these commensals is essential to prevent chronic inflammation in skin.
- Tolerance to commensal skin bacteria is preferentially established early in life when a unique population of skin regulatory T cells encounters and responds to antigens produced by these bacteria.
- Improved understanding of how our skin establishes and maintains tolerance to commensal bacteria may lead to therapeutic approaches to prevent and treat inflammatory skin disease.

INTRODUCTION
Commensal Bacteria in Inflammatory Skin Disease

As dermatologists, we routinely diagnose and treat overt cutaneous infections, such as folliculitis or cellulitis, where a discrete pathogen is causative and antibiotics are curative. We are also familiar with autoimmune skin conditions, such as pemphigus or pemphigoid, where an immune response to a self-antigen results in destructive skin inflammation, and treatments aim to limit this via immunosuppression. However, we also care for many patients with inflammatory skin disorders that are neither infectious nor autoimmune by classical definitions. A few examples of these include atopic dermatitis, acne vulgaris, and hidradenitis suppurativa. Although the pathogenesis of these diseases is clearly multifactorial, it is likely that immune responses directed at the cutaneous microbiota help to drive inflammation (**Fig. 1**).[1]

In atopic dermatitis, hereditary defects in skin barrier integrity or host immunity can confer disease susceptibility, perhaps by driving altered responses to skin bacteria.[2] Flares are accompanied by an increase in the cutaneous burden of *Staphylococcus aureus* and *Staphylococcus epidermidis*.[3] In acne vulgaris, age of onset coincides with a shift in composition of the skin microbiome.[4] As sebaceous activity increases, the proportion of *Propionibacterium acnes* on healthy skin increases. The presence of *P acnes* alone is not sufficient to cause disease, but sequencing of *P acnes* isolates from acne lesions versus healthy skin has revealed a distinct subset of disease-associated strains.[5] In hidradenitis suppurativa, patients suffer from skin lesions that share many clinical features with infectious furuncles or abscesses. However, microbiological studies of hidradenitis lesions consistently demonstrate altered bacterial communities in which commensal strains from skin or other mucosal body sites predominate over skin pathogens.[6] Thus, in these conditions the presence of a single bacterial strain is not sufficient to initiate disease. Rather, shifts in skin flora composition, accompanied by an altered immune response to these bacteria in susceptible hosts likely trigger pathogenic inflammation.[7]

Department of Dermatology, University of California, San Francisco, 1701 Divisadero Street, 3rd Floor, San Francisco, CA 94115, USA
E-mail address: tiffany.scharschmidt@ucsf.edu

Dermatol Clin 35 (2017) 1–9
http://dx.doi.org/10.1016/j.det.2016.07.007
0733-8635/17/© 2016 Elsevier Inc. All rights reserved.

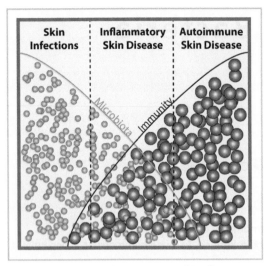

| Skin Infections | Inflammatory Skin Disease | Autoimmune Skin Disease |

Fig. 1. Microbiota and immunity in skin disease. Our skin's microbiota and immune system contribute to the pathogenesis of many diseases. Frank skin infections by pathogens lie at 1 end of the spectrum; whereas, autoimmune noninfectious conditions resulting from aberrant immune responses to self-antigens lie at the other. The pathogenesis of many inflammatory skin diseases fall between these extremes, with important roles for both microbiota and the resulting immune response.

Present treatment for these inflammatory skin diseases include antibiotics; that is, a sledgehammer to reduce the burden of skin flora and topical or systemic immunosuppressive agents to blunt the resulting immune response. Understanding how our cutaneous immune system regulates inflammation directed against skin microbes will provide additional insight into the pathogenesis of these conditions and may open new opportunities to optimize host–microbe interactions for therapeutic benefit.

CONTENT

Skin Commensal Bacteria: How Do We Keep the Peace?

Billions of bacteria, viruses, and fungi reside on our skin's surface and in adenexal structures.[8] Langerhans cells can protrude through tight junctions to capture bacterial antigens on the skin's surface, and bacterial components have even been identified deep in the dermis.[9] This close proximity enables a constant dialogue between these commensals and our immune system. The presence of bacteria augments the skin's production of antimicrobial peptides and alters the number and function of skin-resident lymphocytes.[10,11] Indeed, individual strains of commensal bacteria, such as S epidermidis and P acnes, elicit distinct profiles

of cytokine production by skin lymphocytes, demonstrating that the composition of our skin flora can influence the tissue's immunologic "tone."[12]

A primary function of our immune system is to protect us from infections by recognizing and responding to microbial antigens. The observation that our immune system is clearly responding to our skin commensal bacteria on an ongoing basis leaves us with a fundamental question that has important implications for normal skin biology and the pathogenesis of inflammatory skin disease. Why do our commensal bacteria not elicit chronic inflammation in healthy skin?

Regulatory T Cells: Our Immunologic Peacekeepers

Our immune system is constantly making decisions about whether and how to respond to antigens it encounters. Most of these antigens are our own "self" antigens. Although many self-reactive T cells are deleted during development in the thymus, others escape and their response must be regulated locally in the tissues where these antigens reside. Regulatory T cells (Tregs), a CD4[+] T-cell subset, play a central role in this process of immune regulation or tolerance.[13] As evidence of this, deficiency in the number or function of Tregs leads to autoimmune disease and inflammation in skin and other tissues.[14,15]

Our commensal microbes are in many ways an extension of our human "self"—not only do we rely on them for critical metabolic functions but, as noted, commensal antigens are pervasive at our body surfaces. Commensal bacteria in our gut have been shown to augment the number and function of Tregs in the intestinal lamina propria,[16,17] and gut inflammation seen in the absence of Tregs is directed in part toward luminal microbiota.[18] The skin, like the gut, has a significant population of tissue-resident Tregs.[19] However, the role of these Tregs in immune tolerance to skin bacteria was unexplored until recently.

A Good (Immunologic) Relationship Gets off on the Right Foot

The beginning of life represents a critical window of immune maturation in which our immune system is trained to recognize self and non-self. Neonates, especially in prematurity, are more susceptible to certain infections. Previously this was thought to be because of the "immaturity" of their immune systems. Instead, recent evidence suggests that the immune response in this early stage of life is not underdeveloped but rather carefully designed to promote tolerogenic responses.[20,21] In particular, Tregs generated early in life have a unique propensity to protect tissues from autoimmune attack.[22] Likely this is an adaptive feature to limit potentially damaging immune responses to many new antigens (self and non-self) that the immune system encounters in this developmental window. Colonization by commensal microbiota also occurs at the beginning of life,[23] suggesting that perhaps we educate our immune system to recognize and tolerate commensal microbes at the same time as we learn to tolerate our own antigens.

A New Model to Track Commensal-Specific T Cells and Tolerance

We set out to dissect mechanisms that help us to regulate our adaptive immune response to skin commensal bacteria. T cells have unique surface T-cell receptors, enabling each cell to recognize and respond to a specific antigen. Studying tolerance necessitates isolating just those T cells capable of responding to that antigen and tracking their response in the context of a broad immune repertoire. Tools have not yet been developed to identify and study individual T cells that respond to native antigens made by skin commensal bacteria. Thus, we engineered a skin commensal to express a foreign peptide for which tools are available to track the antigen-specific response (Fig. 2).[24]

We chose to examine the immune response to *S epidermidis*, a prevalent commensal on human skin that also functions as a commensal in mice,

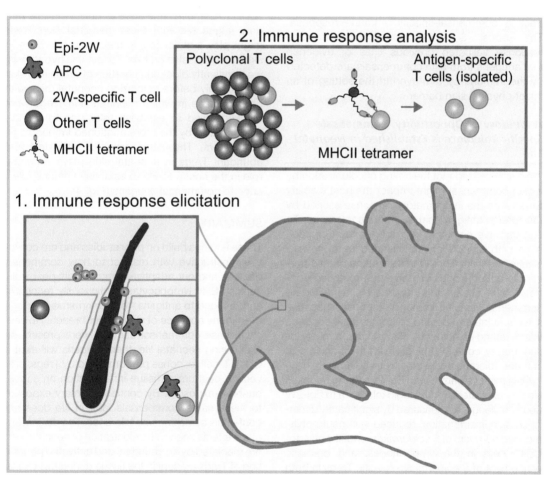

Fig. 2. Tracking commensal-specific immune responses. Studying the adaptive immune response to a skin commensal requires the ability to isolate T cells responding to commensal antigens from a mixed cell population. To create such a system, we engineered the bacteria *Staphylococcus epidermidis* to express a small peptide antigen, 2W (Epi-2W). In mice colonized with Epi-2W, antigen-presenting cells (APC) are able to internalize the 2W antigen and present it to T cells expressing receptors specific for this antigen. To identify and study this commensal-specific immune response, T cells are isolated from Epi-2W–colonized mice and incubated with a tetramer of major histocompatibility complex class II (MHC II) molecules loaded with the 2W peptide. Commensal-specific CD4$^+$ T cells recognizing 2W preferentially bind to this tetramer allowing isolation and characterization of this commensal-specific T-cell population by flow cytometry.

and engineered it to express the foreign peptide, 2W (Epi-2W). A subset of CD4$^+$ T cells in wild-type mice are capable of responding to 2W.[25] These cells can be isolated and studied by flow cytometry using a major histocompatibility complex class II tetramer that binds to the T-cell receptor unique to these cells.[26]

We colonized the skin surface of adult wild-type mice with Epi-2W and examined total inflammation in the skin tissue as well as the 2W-specific (ie, S epidermidis-specific) CD4$^+$ T cells in these animals. After skin colonization, we observed expansion of S epidermidis-specific T cells in both skin-draining lymph nodes and spleen without any accompanying skin inflammation. This suggested that we had successfully created a model of skin commensalism in which we could track a commensal-specific immune response. The robust S epidermidis–specific immune response validated previous lines of evidence that antigens from skin commensals are detected by the immune system even in the setting of an intact physical skin barrier.

A Window of Opportunity: Commensal-Specific Tolerance Is Established in Neonatal Life

We hypothesized that the timing of colonization by a skin commensal might impact the host's ability to regulate the inflammatory response elicited by this foreign antigen, that is, immune tolerance. To test this, we colonized skin of neonatal or adult mice with Epi-2W and challenged them several weeks later with Epi-2W in the setting of mild barrier disruption alongside naïve age-matched controls. We chose this approach to elucidate commensal-specific immune responses because it recapitulates exposure to commensal antigens in the setting of incidental skin trauma, a mildly inflammatory context during which mechanisms of immune tolerance would need to be active.

Only mice colonized with Epi-2W during neonatal life demonstrated immunologic tolerance to Epi-2W upon challenge, as measured by significantly diminished skin inflammation, reduced skin neutrophils, reduced numbers of S epidermidis–specific effector CD4$^+$ cells in the lymph nodes, and dramatic enrichment of S epidermidis–specific Tregs in both skin and lymph nodes. These results demonstrate that colonization of neonatal but not adult skin results in commensal-specific T-cell tolerance (**Fig. 3**).

Peacekeepers Get There Early: A Wave of Regulatory T Cells in Developing Skin

This observation that the timing of exposure to a commensal bacteria influences the ability to establish tolerance prompted us to explore how neonatal and adult skin differ with respect to the resident immune cell populations. Comprehensive immunologic examination of neonatal skin revealed that a unique population of Tregs enters skin during the second week of life. These neonatal skin Tregs are more activated and abundant than their adult counterparts, constitute the majority of T cells in skin during this key developmental window, and are unique to the skin versus another key barrier site, the gut.

Neonatal Skin Regulatory T Cells: Critical Players at the Peacekeeping Table

The abrupt accumulation of activated Tregs in neonatal skin in conjunction with the preferential ability to establish tolerance to Epi-2W in this window suggested that these neonatal skin Tregs might play a major role in mediating tolerance to skin commensal microbes. To test this hypothesis, we transiently blocked migration of Tregs into skin immediately before colonizing neonatal mice with Epi-2W. Mice in which neonatal skin Tregs were blocked failed to establish tolerance to Epi-2W as measured by the aforementioned immunologic parameters. Thus, this wave of activated and abundant Tregs in neonatal skin plays a central role in the host's ability to establish immune tolerance to commensal antigens (**Fig. 4**).

SUMMARY

These findings build on prior studies and are collectively instructive with respect to how commensal bacteria and our adaptive immune cells peacefully coexist. Skin lymphocytes continuously recognize and respond to antigens from commensal bacteria even in the absence of skin barrier breach. However, if these commensal bacteria were present on skin during neonatal life, their antigens will elicit a CD4$^+$ T-cell response predominated by Tregs, preventing destructive tissue inflammation on subsequent re-exposure. By contrast, primary exposure to these same commensals later in life does not confer this same immune tolerance. The distinct immune effects seen with colonization of neonatal skin are mediated by an abundant and activated population of Tregs present in the tissue during this critical developmental window.[24] Below we highlight some of the questions raised by our work and discuss how these may inform our understanding and treatment of patients with inflammatory skin disease (**Fig. 5**).

From Mice to Men

There are important differences between the adaptive immune system in young humans and

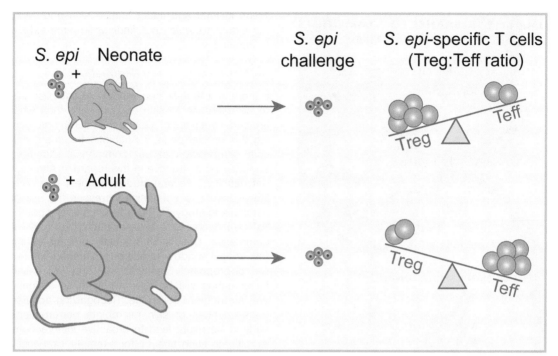

Fig. 3. Immune tolerance to commensals is established early in life. We colonized either neonatal or adult mice with Epi-2W and then several weeks later challenged them again with the bacteria in the setting of skin barrier breach. After this challenge, we characterized the population of commensal-specific T cells as well as the degree of skin inflammation. Epi-2W colonization of neonates resulted in a population of commensal-specific CD4+ T cells that was dominated by T regulatory cells (Tregs). In contrast, Epi-2W colonization of adults led to a predominance of T effectors (Teff) rather than Treg CD4+ T cells. Moreover, neonatal but not adult Epi-2W colonization was protective against skin inflammation upon challenge. Taken together these results show that immune tolerance to skin commensal bacteria is preferentially established early in life. *S. epi, Staphylococcus epidermidis.*

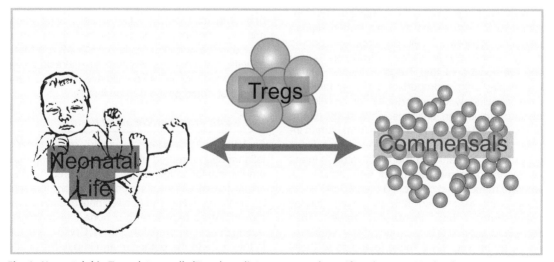

Fig. 4. Neonatal skin T regulatory cells (Tregs) mediate commensal-specific tolerance. Mechanisms to promote immune tolerance to skin commensal bacteria are preferentially active in neonatal life. During this period, a population of abundant and activated Tregs enters skin. This Treg population plays a critical role in establishing tolerance to these commensal bacteria.

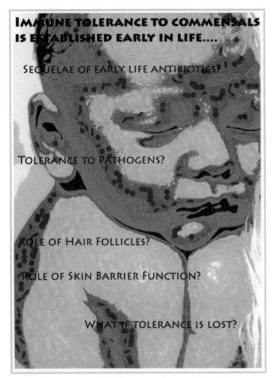

Fig. 5. Commensal-specific immune tolerance: what lies ahead? Recognizing that commensal-specific immune tolerance is established preferentially in early life raises many intriguing questions of relevance to our patients. How do antibiotics, pathogenic microbes, skin barrier function, or hair follicles affect the development of tolerance in neonatal skin and how is it maintained or lost later in life? Answering these and other questions will inform our understanding of cutaneous host–commensal dialogue.

young mice. For example, the immune system develops to a large extent in utero during human gestation, whereas T-cell development occurs largely postnatally in mice.[21] However, recent work demonstrates that Tregs in human infants also display unique properties and may facilitate a similar window of opportunity for developing tolerance to foreign antigens. One study examining lymphoid and mucosal tissue from human infants, adolescents, and adults found that Tregs were more abundant and more activated in infant tissues as compared with those from adults.[27] A separate randomized controlled trial of 640 human infants with heightened risk of peanut allergy demonstrated that increased rather than decreased exposure to peanut protein was protective by helping to establish tolerance to these antigens.[28] These studies suggest that fundamental aspects of our findings may extend to the human biology. Nonetheless, more work is required to define the timing and activation of

Tregs in fetal and infant human skin and verify the extent to which our findings in mice extend to humans.

Do Not Be Late to the Negotiations

If there is a time-limited window to establish immune tolerance to skin commensals, then what are consequences of altering the microbiome during this crucial period? Antibiotic treatment can shift composition of our commensal skin flora and may be instructive in this regard.[29] Although not definitive, several studies suggest that early life exposure to antibiotics increases the risk of asthma and atopy.[30–32] Our findings offer a potential explanation for this association; that is, if the commensal population normally present during this critical window is altered, tolerance will not be appropriately established and increased inflammation will be seen when these antigens are introduced later in life. Recognizing adverse consequences of skin microbiota perturbations early in life might lead to proactive interventions to mitigate such effects; for example, potentially pairing antibiotics with topical probiotics.

A related but distinct question is whether failure to establish tolerance to a commensal early in life precludes tolerance from ever being established or whether other mechanisms could compensate for this later in life. Although our studies suggest that exposure for 1 to 2 weeks during adulthood was insufficient to limit subsequent inflammatory responses to commensal antigens, colonization over a longer period of time might attenuate inflammation via alternate mechanisms, much like dose-escalating drug exposure protocols used to desensitize allergic individuals who require that drug for therapy.[33] Conversely, once tolerance to a commensal is established in neonates, how durable is this immune response? Are there specific mechanisms required to maintain tolerance throughout life or specific events or interventions that could cause it to be lost?

Can a Foe Masquerade as a Friend?

Evolutionary pressures to avoid overwhelming inflammation directed at self or highly abundance environmental antigens may have favored mechanisms to establish tolerance to antigens present on skin early in life. The Achilles heel of such a system might be exposure to a bona fide pathogen during this developmental window. Could this result in tolerance to the pathogen and impair the host's ability to fight infection by this pathogen later in life?

The complexity of the immune response suggests that answers to these questions are unlikely to be black and white. In the case of an overt infection by a skin pathogen during this developmental window, innate immune signals triggered by skin barrier breach might override the tolerogenic response and instead support an effector T-cell response to clear the pathogen. However, the immunologic outcome is less clear for skin colonization by bacterial pathogens that do not always breach the epidermidis, for example, S aureus. Understanding the consequences of S aureus colonization early in life, especially in individuals with atopic dermatitis, will have important implications for these patients who are prone to recurrent flares of their disease in association with this bacteria.[34]

Host–Commensal Immune Dialogue: A 3-Dimensional Conversation

Spatial as well as temporal aspects of immune cell interactions are critical to shaping the quality of the resulting immune response.[35] Thus far, we have explored how temporal factors may influence our ability to establish tolerance to commensals. Thinking about where this dialogue takes place in the tissue may be equally important.

Cutaneous Tregs localize to hair follicles, where a high burden of commensal bacteria reside.[19,36] The spatial colocalization of these populations may facilitate establishment and maintenance of commensal-specific tolerance. Mutations in genes critical to the structural integrity of the skin barrier, for example, filaggrin, increase permeability of interfollicular skin to exogenous antigens and confer significant risk for atopic dermatitis.[37] If an altered skin barrier directs presentation of commensal antigens away from the hair follicle, it may impair mechanisms that promote establishment of commensal-specific tolerance and result in excessive inflammation directed at these antigens. In acne vulgaris and hidradenitis, skin inflammation tends to be focused around hair follicles. If hair follicles provide a structure facilitating commensal Treg interaction, then physical disruption of this skin niche, as occurs in both these conditions, may impair maintenance of commensal-specific tolerance and lead to increased tissue inflammation directed as these "healthy" microbes.

Commensal Bacteria in Inflammatory Skin Disease: What Lies Ahead?

Understanding that a healthy immune response to commensal bacteria requires interaction between Tregs and these bacterial antigens early in life may eventually impact clinical practice. For example, and as suggested, antibiotic-induced alteration of the skin microbiota during infancy may predispose to inflammation later in life.[32] Although often necessary and life saving, antibiotics should always be used judiciously, especially during this critical developmental window. Recognition of antibiotics' untoward effects on the gut microbiota has increasingly led to the administration of probiotics during or after antibiotic therapy to help rescue and restore the normal gut flora. The same may pertain in the future to skin, where antibiotics might be paired with topical probiotics to mitigate disruption of normal commensals.

It may also be possible to exploit these mechanisms for host–commensal tolerance by establishing tolerance to selected foreign antigens for which immune tolerance would be advantageous. For example, patients lacking certain epidermal proteins may soon be able to benefit from gene replacement therapy. A barrier to success with such treatments is the propensity for adaptive immune responses that target and kill cells expressing these "foreign" proteins or those associated with vectors used for gene delivery.[38] Genetic conditions affecting the skin that might benefit from gene replacement are often diagnosed at birth or soon thereafter, allowing us a window of opportunity for commensal-driven expression of these foreign antigens that might prime the patient's immune system for tolerance upon subsequent replacement therapy.

Although there is much yet to learn, harnessing mechanisms that regulate immune responses to commensal bacteria may eventually improve therapy for complex inflammatory skin disorders, such as atopic dermatitis, acne vulgaris or hidradenitis suppurativa. This will require not only characterizing changes in microbiota composition associated with inflammatory skin disease but also determining the extent to which adaptive immune responses in the tissue are directed against and driven by microbial antigens. Although not an easy task with tools currently available, emerging technologies enabling analysis of single cells from patient's skin lesions and engineering of chimeric antigen receptor T cells to study effects of commensal-specific T cells in model systems may render these questions tractable.[39,40] Empowered with this knowledge as well as basic research examining mechanisms required to maintain or reestablish tolerance to commensals later in life, we may start to identify and reverse patterns that drive disease pathogenesis. The many as yet unanswered questions pertaining to host–microbe immunobiology make this a rich and exciting field for future investigation and one that has the potential to eventually shift our understanding of and approach to inflammatory skin disease.

REFERENCES

1. Belkaid Y, Segre JA. Dialogue between skin microbiota and immunity. Science 2014;346(6212):954–9.

2. Hoffjan S, Stemmler S. Unravelling the complex genetic background of atopic dermatitis: from genetic association results towards novel therapeutic strategies. Arch Dermatol Res 2015;307(8):659–70.

3. Kong HH, Oh J, Deming C, et al. Temporal shifts in the skin microbiome associated with disease flares and treatment in children with atopic dermatitis. Genome Res 2012;22(5):850–9.

4. Oh J, Conlan S, Polley EC, et al. Shifts in human skin and nares microbiota of healthy children and adults. Genome Med 2012;4(10):77.

5. Fitz-Gibbon S, Tomida S, Chiu B-H, et al. Propionibacterium acnes strain populations in the human skin microbiome associated with acne. J Invest Dermatol 2013;133(9):2152–60.

6. Nikolakis G, Join-Lambert O, Karagiannidis I, et al. Bacteriology of hidradenitis suppurativa/acne inversa: a review. J Am Acad Dermatol 2015; 73(5 Suppl 1):S12–8.

7. Scharschmidt TC, Fischbach MA. What lives on our skin: ecology, genomics and therapeutic opportunities of the skin microbiome. Drug Discov Today Dis Mech 2013;10(3–4).

8. Oh J, Byrd AL, Deming C, et al. Biogeography and individuality shape function in the human skin metagenome. Nature 2014;514(7520):59–64.

9. Kubo A, Nagao K, Yokouchi M, et al. External antigen uptake by Langerhans cells with reorganization of epidermal tight junction barriers. J Exp Med 2009; 206(13):2937–46.

10. Lai Y, Cogen AL, Radek KA, et al. Activation of TLR2 by a small molecule produced by staphylococcus epidermidis increases antimicrobial defense against bacterial skin infections. J Invest Dermatol 2011; 130(9):2211–21.

11. Naik S, Bouladoux N, Wilhelm C, et al. Compartmentalized control of skin immunity by resident commensals. Science 2012;337(6098):1115–9.

12. Naik S, Bouladoux N, Linehan JL, et al. Commensal-dendritic-cell interaction specifies a unique protective skin immune signature. Nature 2015;520(7545): 104–8.

13. Gratz IK, Rosenblum MD, Abbas AK. The life of regulatory T cells. Ann N Y Acad Sci 2013; 1283(1):8–12.

14. Brunkow ME, Jeffery EW, Hjerrild KA, et al. Disruption of a new forkhead/winged-helix protein, scurfin, results in the fatal lymphoproliferative disorder of the scurfy mouse. Nat Genet 2001;27(1):68–73.

15. Wildin RS, Ramsdell F, Peake J, et al. X-linked neonatal diabetes mellitus, enteropathy and endocrinopathy syndrome is the human equivalent of mouse scurfy. Nat Genet 2001;27(1):18–20.

16. Atarashi K, Tanoue T, Shima T, et al. Induction of colonic regulatory T Cells by indigenous clostridium species. Science 2011;331(6015):337–41.

17. Round JL, Mazmanian SK. Inducible Foxp3+ regulatory T-cell development by a commensal bacterium of the intestinal microbiota. Proc Natl Acad Sci U S A 2010;107(27):12204–9.

18. Cahill RJ, Foltz CJ, Fox JG, et al. Inflammatory bowel disease: an immunity-mediated condition triggered by bacterial infection with Helicobacter hepaticus. Infect Immun 1997;65(8):3126–31.

19. Sanchez Rodriguez R, Pauli ML, Neuhaus IM, et al. Memory regulatory T cells reside in human skin. J Clin Invest 2014;124(3):1027–36.

20. Elahi S, Ertelt JM, Kinder JM, et al. Immunosuppressive CD71+ erythroid cells compromise neonatal host defence against infection. Nature 2013; 504(7478):158–62.

21. Mold JE, McCune JM. Immunological tolerance during fetal development: from mouse to man. Adv Immunol 2012;115:73–111.

22. Yang S, Fujikado N, Kolodin D, et al. Regulatory T cells generated early in life play a distinct role in maintaining self-tolerance. Science 2015; 348(6234):589–94.

23. Dominguez-Bello MG, Costello EK, Contreras M, et al. Delivery mode shapes the acquisition and structure of the initial microbiota across multiple body habitats in newborns. Proc Natl Acad Sci U S A 2010;107(26):11971–5.

24. Scharschmidt TC, Vasquez KS, Truong H-A, et al. A wave of regulatory T cells into neonatal skin mediates tolerance to commensal microbes. Immunity 2015;43(5):1011–21.

25. Moon JJ, Chu HH, Pepper M, et al. Naive CD4(+) T cell frequency varies for different epitopes and predicts repertoire diversity and response magnitude. Immunity 2007;27(2):203–13.

26. Moon JJ, Chu HH, Hataye J, et al. Tracking epitope-specific T cells. Nat Protoc 2009;4(4):565–81.

27. Thome JJC, Bickham KL, Ohmura Y, et al. Early-life compartmentalization of human T cell differentiation and regulatory function in mucosal and lymphoid tissues. Nat Med 2015;22(1):72–7.

28. Toit Du G, Roberts G, Sayre PH, et al. Randomized trial of peanut consumption in infants at risk for peanut allergy. N Engl J Med 2015;372(9): 803–13.

29. Marples RR, Kligman AM. Ecological effects of oral antibiotics on the microflora of human skin. Arch Dermatol 1971;103(2):148–53.

30. Russell SL, Gold MJ, Hartmann M, et al. Early life antibiotic-driven changes in microbiota enhance susceptibility to allergic asthma. EMBO Rep 2012; 13(5):440–7.

31. McKeever TM, Lewis SA, Smith C, et al. Early exposure to infections and antibiotics and the incidence

of allergic disease: a birth cohort study with the west midlands general practice research database. J Allergy Clin Immunol 2002;109(1):43–50.

32. Willing BP, Russell SL, Finlay BB. Shifting the balance: antibiotic effects on host–microbiota mutualism. Nat Rev Microbiol 2011;9(4):233–43.

33. Akdis CA, Akdis M. Mechanisms of allergen-specific immunotherapy. J Allergy Clin Immunol 2011;127(1): 18–27.

34. Nagao K, Segre JA. "Bringing Up Baby" to tolerate germs. Immunity 2015;43(5):842–4.

35. Qi H, Kastenmüller W, Germain RN. Spatiotemporal basis of innate and adaptive immunity in secondary lymphoid tissue*. Annu Rev Cell Dev Biol 2014; 30(1):141–67.

36. Gratz IK, Truong H-A, Yang SH-Y, et al. Cutting edge: memory regulatory t cells require IL-7 and not IL-2 for their maintenance in peripheral tissues. J Immunol 2013;190(9):4483–7.

37. Scharschmidt TC, Man M-Q, Hatano Y, et al. Filaggrin deficiency confers a paracellular barrier abnormality that reduces inflammatory thresholds to irritants and haptens. J Allergy Clin Immunol 2009; 124(3):496–506, 506.e1–6.

38. Wu T-L, Ertl HCJ. Immune barriers to successful gene therapy. Trends Mol Med 2009;15(1):32–9.

39. Curran KJ, Pegram HJ, Brentjens RJ. Chimeric antigen receptors for T cell immunotherapy: current understanding and future directions. J Gene Med 2012;14(6):405–15.

40. Shapiro E, Biezuner T, Linnarsson S. Single-cell sequencing-based technologies will revolutionize whole-organism science. Nat Rev Genet 2013; 14(9):618–30.

Current Status of Dedicator of Cytokinesis-Associated Immunodeficiency DOCK8 and DOCK2

Dimana Dimitrova, MD[a], Alexandra F. Freeman, MD[b],*

KEYWORDS

- Immunodeficiency • Dedicator of cytokinesis 8 • Dedicator of cytokinesis 2 • Atopic dermatitis
- Cutaneous viral infection • Malignancy

KEY POINTS

- DOCK8 deficiency is an autosomal recessive hyper–immunoglobulin E syndrome associated with atopy, recurrent sinopulmonary and cutaneous viral infections, and malignancies.
- The DOCK8 protein plays an important role in cytoskeletal organization, impacting dendritic cell transmigration.
- DOCK8 deficiency leads to persistence of B cells in germinal centers, early T-cell death, and lowered natural killler cell cytotoxicity.
- DOCK2 deficiency has been recently described in several patients with early-onset invasive bacterial and viral infections.

INTRODUCTION

Dedicator of cytokinesis 8 (DOCK8) deficiency is an autosomal recessive combined immunodeficiency syndrome characterized by recurrent sinopulmonary and cutaneous viral infections, as well as an increased immunoglobulin (Ig)E level and atopy. Although patients with an autosomal recessive variant of hyper-IgE syndrome had been described as early as 2004, a genetic basis involving bi-allelic mutations often with large deletions was not established until 2009.[1–3] In the intervening years, definitive treatment with early hematopoietic stem cell transplantation (HSCT) has gained prominence, and advances have been made in understanding the functions of DOCK8 in dendritic cell and lymphocyte activity. Recently, another syndrome with differing phenotype but similar immunopathogenic basis, dedicator of cytokinesis 2 (DOCK2) deficiency, has been described.[4]

CLINICAL PRESENTATION OF DEDICATOR OF CYTOKINESIS 8 DEFICIENCY
Atopy

Patients with DOCK8 deficiency demonstrate atopy early on. Nearly all patients exhibit atopic dermatitis (AD), which ranges from mild to very severe and difficult to treat (**Fig. 1**). Unlike patients with autosomal dominant hyper-IgE syndrome from Signal transducer and activator of transcription 3 (STAT3)

Neither author has any commercial or financial conflicts of interest.

[a] Experimental Transplantation and Immunology Branch, National Cancer Institute, National Institutes of Health, 10 Center Drive, Bethesda, MD 20892, USA; [b] Laboratory of Clinical Infectious Diseases, National Institute of Allergy and Infectious Diseases, National Institutes of Health, 10 Center Drive, Bethesda, MD 20892, USA
* Corresponding author. NIH Building 10 Room 12C103, Bethesda, MD 20892.
E-mail address: freemaal@mail.nih.gov

Dermatol Clin 35 (2017) 11–19
http://dx.doi.org/10.1016/j.det.2016.07.002
0733-8635/17/Published by Elsevier Inc.

Abbreviations and acronyms	
Cdc42	G protein activated by DOCK guanine exchange factors.
DOCK2	Dedicator of cytokinesis 2, one of a class of guanine nucleotide exchange factors whose role is to activate the G protein Rac.
DOCK8	Dedicator of cytokinesis 8, one of a class of guanine nucleotide exchange factors whose role is to activate G proteins such as Rac and Cdc42. Deficiency leads to impaired cytoskeletal organization and a phenotype of combined immunodeficiency with eczema, elevated IgE, and malignancy.
HSCT	Hematopoietic stem cell transplantation, a treatment for primary immunodeficiencies that result from genetic defects in hematopoietic cells.
ICAM-1	Intercellular adhesion molecule 1, a ligand for LFA-1 necessary for leukocyte endothelial transmigration.
LFA-1	Lymphocyte function–associated antigen 1, binds to ICAM-1 and functions as an adhesion molecule.
MST1	Macrophage-stimulating 1 (also known as STK4). Deficiency results in a rare form of immunodeficiency with a phenotype similar to DOCK8 deficiency.
MyD88	Myeloid differentiation primary response 88, a protein used by Toll-like receptors to activate the transcription factor NF-κB.
PGM3	Phosphoglucomutase 3, which mediates glycosylation. Deficiency results in a phenotype of severe atopy, hypergammaglobulinemia, leukopenia, and developmental delay.
Rac	G protein activated by DOCK guanine exchange factors.
Rho GTPase	G protein such as Cdc42 and Rac, activated by DOCK guanine exchange factors. These proteins regulate various aspects of cytoskeletal dynamics.
STAT3	Signal transducer and activator of transcription 3, a transcription factor. Deficiency leads to autosomal dominant hyper-IgE syndrome.
TLR9	Toll-like receptor 9, important for activation of innate immunity via MyD88.
Tyk2	Tyrosine kinase 2, a protein involved in IL-10 and IFN-α signaling. Deficiency has been associated with a variable phenotype that includes susceptibility to mycobacterial infection.
WAS	Wiskott-Aldrich syndrome is a rare X-linked recessive disease classically characterized by a triad of recurrent sinopulmonary infections, eczema, and thrombocytopenia with small platelets. Many patients do not exhibit the classic triad and may have autoimmune disease among other manifestations.
WASp	Wiskott-Aldrich syndrome protein, a protein that coordinates cytoskeletal reorganization. Deficiency leads to WAS.

mutations, many have food allergies with anaphylaxis, as well as asthma. Eosinophilic esophagitis also has been seen with increased frequency.[3,5–7]

Infections

Cellulitis and skin abscesses are common, as is mucocutaneous candidiasis. There is a striking susceptibility to cutaneous infections by viruses, such as human papillomavirus (HPV) leading to widespread and recalcitrant warts, extensive and disfiguring molluscum contagiosum, herpes simplex virus (HSV) with recurrent or persistent lesions or herpes keratitis, and varicella zoster virus (VZV) with severe primary infection or recurrent zoster (**Fig. 2**). Chronic Epstein-Barr virus (EBV) viremia is frequent, and may be associated with transformation to malignancy. Interestingly, severe systemic viral infections are less common, although several patients have suffered from cytomegalovirus (CMV) disease, encephalitis, and progressive multifocal leukoencephalopathy.[3,5–7]

Most patients have a history of recurrent sinusitis and otitis media requiring tympanostomy tubes. Most also have had multiple pneumonias, with development of bronchiectasis in more than a third but infrequent pneumatocele formation (**Fig. 3**).[3,5–7]

Malignancy

Increased risk of neoplasms, especially hematological and epithelial, is an important feature of DOCK8 deficiency, and malignancy is often particularly aggressive and has early onset. In one large cohort of 136 patients, 17% of patients were diagnosed with malignancy at a median age of 12 years.[6] Malignancy most frequently arises from poor control of viruses including squamous cell carcinomas from HPV infection and EBV-related lymphomas. Microcystic adnexal carcinoma, aggressive cutaneous T-cell lymphoma, and diffuse large B-cell lymphoma have been described.[3,8] Of note, not all tumors have been associated with viral infection.

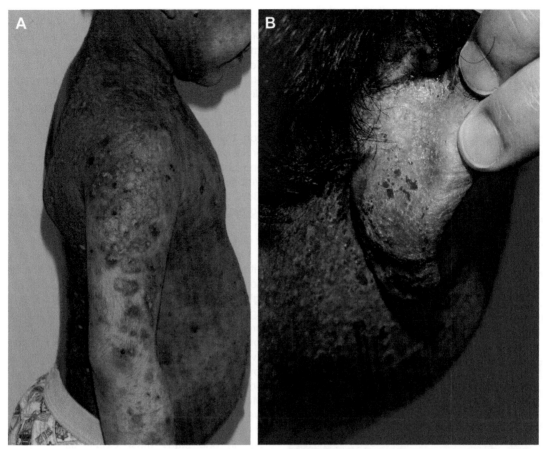

Fig. 1. (*A*, *B*) Chronic severe eczematous dermatitis in a 6-year-old boy with DOCK8 deficiency.

Other Clinical Manifestations

Vascular abnormalities have been recognized in more than 10% of patients in 2 recently described large cohorts (Fig. 4). Cerebral aneurysms and stenosis are seen, and have been associated with stroke. Vaccine strain varicella was identified as the etiologic agent in one case, but in others an infectious has not been identified. Aortic aneurysm and abdominal arterial vasculitis also have been described, without known etiology. Autoimmunity

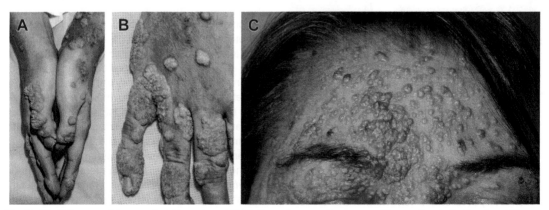

Fig. 2. (*A*, *B*) Large, widespread warts as a manifestation of severe human papilloma virus infection in a 15-year-old girl with DOCK8 deficiency. (*C*) Extensive molluscum contagiosum in a patient with DOCK8 deficiency.

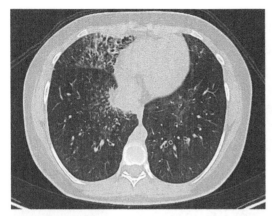

Fig. 3. Computed tomography of the chest of a 15-year-old girl with DOCK8 deficiency shows right middle lobe bronchiectasis with thickened bronchial walls.

rarely has manifested in other forms, such as hemolytic anemia.[6,7] Liver disease, both associated with and without cryptosporidia has been described as well, and can be quite significant, leading to liver transplantation.[9,10]

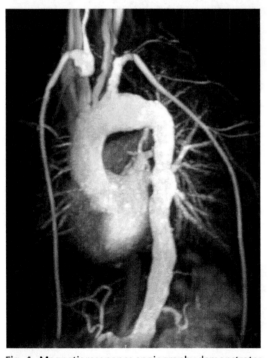

Fig. 4. Magnetic resonance angiography demonstrates vasculopathy in a 19-year-old patient with DOCK8 deficiency. Shown are a dilated ascending and transverse thoracic aorta with diffuse irregularity and foci of narrowing in the descending aorta. Other findings (not shown) included narrowing at the bifurcation of the right brachial cephalic artery, dilatation of the right subclavian artery at its origin, narrowing of the left common carotid, narrowing of the common iliacs, and narrowing of the right external iliac artery.

Laboratory Features

DOCK8 deficiency is a combined T-cell and B-cell immunodeficiency. In the initial cohort of patients described by Zhang and colleagues,[3] all were noted to have normal neutrophils and monocytes. Ninety percent had low total T cells and CD8+ T cells, and all had low CD4+ T cells; 36% had low B and 60% low natural killer (NK) cells. In addition, there was poor CD8+ but not CD4+ T-cell proliferation in response to stimulation. Engelhardt and colleagues[2] observed lower rates of T-cell lymphopenia in their 2009 and 2015 cohorts (38% and 27%, respectively), whereas Aydin and colleagues[6] observed low total lymphocyte counts in 20% of patients but low total T cells and CD4+ T cells in nearly half of patients.[7]

Elevated IgE and eosinophilia were nearly ubiquitous. Consistently, IgG levels were usually normal or elevated, IgA levels were variable, and IgM levels tended to be low and to decline with age.[6] Vaccine responses to polysaccharide and protein antigens were variable, but the patients followed by Zhang and colleagues[3] showed protective titers to rubella and VZV. Half of patients had low or absent specific antibody responses to pneumococcus, diphtheria, tetanus, or *Candida*.[7] Memory B cells in patients with DOCK8 deficiency were near absent, as were switched memory B cells.[7,11] Memory T-cell numbers were variable, but in one study most CD8+ cells had an exhausted CD45RA+/CCR7− phenotype.[7,12] Caracciolo and colleagues[11] noted low numbers of naïve and recent thymic emigrant T lymphocytes, along with Th2 skewing. This is consistent with low T-cell receptor excision circles in 3 children with DOCK8 deficiency, a finding with ramifications for potential early detection of this disease.[13]

Making the Diagnosis

Given the potential for severe infection and malignancy, it is important to recognize DOCK8 deficiency before development of serious complications whenever possible. Diagnosis may be difficult, and, particularly in infants and young children, early presentation may significantly overlap with severe AD in both laboratory and clinical features. Genetic sequencing is key to making the diagnosis, but the expense makes this prohibitive for screening. Thus, several groups have sought to identify markers that can clue in the clinician to an underlying monogenetic disorder. Furthermore, distinguishing features of different monogenetic hyper-IgE syndromes on presentation is important for targeting subsequent evaluations.

When compared with patients with severe AD, patients with DOCK8 deficiency were more likely to have low total T cells, low CD4+ T cells, and decreased naïve CD8+ T cells in one small study. Total B lymphocyte numbers did not differ significantly between the 2 groups, but subsets revealed decreased memory and increased naïve and transitional B cells in the patients with DOCK8 deficiency.[14]

When examining IgE-sensitization patterns in AD, STAT3 deficiency, and DOCK8 deficiency, Boos and colleagues[15] found that patients with AD had the highest ratios of aeroallergen-specific IgE to total IgE, whereas patients with DOCK8 deficiency showed the highest serum-specific IgE against food antigens, followed by patients with AD.

Using the hyper-IgE syndrome scoring system developed by the National Institutes of Health, Engelhardt and colleagues[7] compared clinical and laboratory scoring for DOCK8 and STAT3 patients and identified several objective features that were helpful in distinguishing the 2 syndromes: parenchymal lung abnormalities, retained primary teeth, and minor trauma fractures were deemed most consistent with STAT3 deficiency.[16] Characteristic facies was also significantly associated with STAT3 deficiency but was considered a subjective assessment. By assigning negative points to the 3 features and adding points based on absolute eosinophil count and frequency of sinus and ear infections, the group developed a DOCK8 score that appears promising but has yet to be validated.[7]

Another study featured long-term follow-up of biomarker trends in individual patients with DOCK8 deficiency and STAT3 deficiency. Patients with DOCK8 deficiency demonstrated consistently lower total, CD4+, and CD8+ T-cell numbers but normal Th17 cells as opposed to low Th17 cell but otherwise normal numbers of T cells in patients with STAT3 deficiency. In terms of clinical characteristics, the investigators suggested that a history of recurrent viral infections, bronchial hyperreactivity, food allergies, and consanguinity should prompt greater concern for DOCK8 deficiency.[17]

In addition to severe AD and STAT3 deficiency, the differential diagnosis for a patient with AD, elevated IgE, and recurrent infections includes several other genetic disorders.

- Wiskott-Aldrich syndrome (WAS) is characterized by T-cell lymphopenia, poor lymphocyte proliferation, impaired NK cytotoxicity, autoimmunity, and malignancy. The WAS protein (WASp) coordinates cytoskeletal reorganization downstream from DOCK8, which accounts for some overlap in phenotype, including recurrent bacterial and viral infections, eczema, and

vascular abnormalities. Distinguishing features of WAS include X-linked inheritance and microthrombocytopenia.[18]
- Phosphoglucomutase 3 (PGM3) deficiency, a congenital disorder of glycosylation, has been recently identified in patients who, in addition to severe atopy and hypergammaglobulinemia, usually have lymphopenia and neutropenia. Developmental delay or neurologic impairment is common.[19]
- Omenn syndrome is a form of severe combined immunodeficiency associated with several different genetic defects. Severe erythroderma and exfoliative dermatitis are evident in early infancy, along with elevated IgE, infections, lymphadenopathy, and hepatosplenomegaly.[20]
- STK4 or Macrophage-Stimulating 1 (MST1) deficiency, discovered within the past few years, has a phenotype similar to DOCK8 deficiency, with cutaneous viral, bacterial, and fungal infections, recurrent respiratory infections, and CD4 lymphopenia. AD seems to be milder, and IgG and IgA are elevated as well as IgE. Cardiac anomalies have been noted in multiple patients.[21]
- Tyk2 deficiency was described in 2006 in a patient with elevated IgE, AD, recurrent skin staphylococcal abscesses, and mycobacterial infection. However, recently, 7 new patients with Tyk2 deficiency were identified, all with normal IgE, calling into question the classification of Tyk2 deficiency as a hyper-IgE syndrome.[22]

FUNCTIONS OF THE DEDICATOR OF CYTOKINESIS 8 PROTEIN

The DOCK8 protein is a member of the DOCK180-related family of atypical guanine nucleotide exchange factors that activate small Rho GTPases, such as Rac and Cdc42.[23,24] These GTPases interact with DOCK8 at actin projections called lamellipodia, which are found at the leading edge of motile cells, such as endothelial cells, neurons, immune cells, and epithelial cells. Early studies suggested DOCK8 as an important player in dynamic actin reorganization because of its accumulation at lamellipodia and its ability to induce formation of vesicles containing filamentous actin.[23] As DOCK8 is highly expressed only in the immune system (and at low levels in nonimmune tissues, such as the placenta, kidney, lung, and pancreas), more recent investigation has shed light on the protein's specific role in the survival and function of dendritic cells (DCs) and lymphocytes.[23,25]

Dendritic Cells

DCs adapt their shape to facilitate ameboid migration through the interstitium. In a DOCK8 knockout mouse model, DCs were unable to crawl through 3-dimensional (3D) fibrillar networks and transmigrate into the lymph node for T-cell priming, due to impaired Cdc42 activation at the leading edge membrane.[26] The peripheral blood of patients with DOCK8 deficiency shows severe deficiency of plasmacytoid dendritic cells and correspondingly low interferon alpha (IFN-α) levels.[27,28]

B LYMPHOCYTES

The B cells of mice lacking DOCK8 cannot develop into marginal zone B cells, survive in germinal centers, and undergo affinity maturation, leading to normal initiation but poor persistence of antibody response after immunization. DOCK8 appears to be required for organization of a B-cell immunologic synapse by recruiting the integrin ligand intercellular adhesion molecule 1 (ICAM-1).[29] In a study of patients with DOCK8 deficiency who showed either poor initial antibody responses to vaccination or poor persistence of protective titers, DOCK8 was shown to function as an adaptor linking Toll-like receptor 9 (TLR9) to myeloid differentiation primary response 88 (MyD88) and downstream signaling pathways to effect B-cell activation.[30]

T, Natural Killer, and Natural Killer T Lymphocytes

Recent studies of DOCK8-deficient mice show a lack of CD4+ T-cell infiltration into HSV-infected skin, associated with poor control of primary cutaneous herpes simplex lesions and increased virus loads.[31]

T-cell lymphopenia is a prominent feature in DOCK8-deficient mice, due to both decreased survival of CD4+ and CD8+ T cells and decreased egress of mature CD4+ T cells from the thymus.[32] Primary T-cell response to infection or immunization is near-normal, but there is poor secondary expansion given reduced survival of memory CD8+ T cells.[12,32] Diminished recruitment of LFA-1 to the CD8+ T cell/DC synapse and delay in the first cell division likely result in impaired generation of long-lived CD8+ T cells.[12]

As mentioned previously, DOCK8 activates Cdc42, which via its effector WASp is necessary for reorganizing the F-actin cytoskeleton in NK and dendritic cells. WASp itself also interacts directly with DOCK8, and WASp function may thus also be reduced in patients with DOCK8 deficiency.[33,34] DOCK8-deficient NK cells show decreased natural and receptor-mediated cytotoxicity, with decreased polarization of LFA-1, F-actin, and cytolytic granules toward the cytotoxic synapse.[33,35]

Zhang and colleagues[36] examined lymphocyte migration through the dermis and found that DOCK8-deficient T and NK cells develop an abnormal shape when moving in confined spaces. In a 3D collagen gel matrix simulating the dermis, the cells were able to move, unlike the nonmotile dendritic cells described by Harada and colleagues,[26] and chemotaxis was not impaired. However, hours later, the cells underwent fragmentation (cytothripsis) and died, suggesting that DOCK8 is essential for coordinating lymphocyte cytoskeletal integrity in this milieu. The early cell death prevents the generation of long-lived skin-resident memory CD8+ T cells, which may explain the preponderance of severe cutaneous viral infections in these patients.

Low NKT cell numbers have been noted in DOCK8-deficient humans, whereas in mice ongoing NKT proliferative and cytokine responses are impaired.[37]

A recent analysis of the cytokine profile of DOCK8 deficiency shows that unstimulated DOCK8-deficient peripheral blood mononuclear cells (PBMCs) secrete higher levels of inflammatory cytokines, such as interferon (IFN)-gamma, interleukin (IL)-1beta, IL-4, and IL-6 as compared with healthy control cells. Interestingly, stimulated PBMCs secreted less IFN-gamma, suggesting impaired Th1 cell function. As Cdc42 is required for IFN-gamma secretion at the immunologic synapse, this finding is consistent with an intrinsic defect secondary to DOCK8 deficiency.[17]

Dedicator of Cytokinesis 8 Expression in Tumors

Many but not all of the malignancies described in DOCK8 deficiency are virus-associated, which has prompted the question of whether the DOCK8 protein may have some intrinsic tumor-suppressive function. Loss of chromosome arm 9p, where the DOCK8 gene is also located, is common in lung cancer.[38] Deletions and other chromosomal alterations encompassing the DOCK8 gene have been associated with lung, gastric, pancreatic, and head and neck squamous cell carcinomas, whereas decreased expression of DOCK8 has been noted in certain lung and liver tumors, as well as in high-grade gliomas.[39–44] However, increased expression of DOCK8 has been noted in a radiosensitive esophageal cancer line and in hepatocellular carcinoma cells, so a consistent role for DOCK8 in tumorigenesis has not emerged.[45,46]

THERAPEUTIC APPROACHES TO DEDICATOR OF CYTOKINESIS 8 DEFICIENCY

Nearly two-thirds of patients receive immunoglobulin replacement therapy, as well as prophylactic antibiotics. Some patients also receive antiviral and antifungal prophylaxis.[6] Even in patients who are otherwise well controlled, HSV lesions, molluscum, and warts may be particularly recalcitrant, disfiguring, and problematic from a quality-of-life standpoint.

Systemic IFN-α 2b therapy, which may act by inhibiting viral replication and activating effector lymphocytes, has yielded dramatic improvement of viral infection in 3 published cases of patients with DOCK8 deficiency.[27,28] However, significant side effects may be associated with IFN-α 2b therapy, and careful monitoring is essential.

Nevertheless, DOCK8 deficiency is associated with significant mortality, mainly due to infection or malignancy. In the cohort described by Engelhardt and colleagues,[7] mean age of death was 9 years and 3 months, whereas Aydin and colleagues[6] report probability of survival of 37% at age 30 years if not transplanted. HSCT has been repeatedly shown to be curative, and more recently is being offered at an early stage. In their initial posttransplant course, patients may have a transient worsening of warts and chronic bacterial pretransplant infections. However, within several months, marked improvement or, more commonly, complete resolution of all skin manifestations has consistently been noted even in patients who previously experienced particularly severe or disfiguring skin disease. Complete immunologic correction has generally been reported, even in several cases of mixed donor chimerism. Two deaths have been described in the literature, one considered transplant-related and one due to *Klebsiella* sepsis in the context of congenital asplenia, and unpublished experience has shown transplant-related mortality in the setting of pretransplant significant end-organ disease.[47–57]

Somatic reversions were identified in 17 patients with DOCK8 deficiency followed at the National Institutes of Health, and these patients demonstrated longer survival and a milder disease course; however, experience with these patients has shown that they may nevertheless have life-threatening complications and require HSCT.[58]

DEDICATOR OF CYTOKINESIS 2 DEFICIENCY

DOCK2, like DOCK8, is a member of the DOCK180 superfamily of proteins. DOCK2-deficient mice were known to have immunologic defects even before DOCK8 deficiency was described in humans. Notable features included T-cell lymphopenia and decreased T-cell proliferation, loss of marginal zone B cells, and decreased myeloid and lymphocyte migration, with the potential for developing hyper-IgE.[25]

Recently, biallelic DOCK 2 mutations were identified in 5 patients with invasive bacterial and viral infections, lymphopenia, and impaired antibody responses.[4] Three of the children were born to consanguineous parents. Infections included recurrent pneumonia, disseminated varicella, *Mycobacterium avium*, mumps meningoencephalitis, and *Klebsiella pneumoniae* sepsis. Unfortunately, only 3 of the patients survived to receive HSCT and attain clinical improvement. Further investigation of the patients' T, B, and NK cells revealed defective chemotaxis, actin polymerization, and NK cell degranulation. Interestingly, viral replication and virus-induced cell death were increased in DOCK2-deficient fibroblasts, and inducing lentiviral-mediated DOCK2 expression in the presence of IFN-α 2b protected the cells. Thus, DOCK2 may impair nonhematopoietic immunity as well. Although some similarities exist between the DOCK2 and DOCK8 deficiency phenotypes, only one of the DOCK2 patients had elevated IgE, and severe eczema and allergies were not prominent features in these patients.

SUMMARY

In the years since DOCK8 deficiency was described, much progress has been made in delineating the phenotype, establishing the role of DOCK8 in leukocyte function, and defining HSCT as a necessary treatment. The phenotype of DOCK2 deficiency in humans remains to be further characterized beyond the index patients.

The growing experience with patients with DOCK8 deficiency highlights the concept that severe skin disease can be an indicator of underlying immunodeficiency, and thus dermatologists may be key to the early diagnosis of this disorder.

REFERENCES

1. Renner ED, Puck JM, Holland SM, et al. Autosomal recessive hyperimmunoglobulin E syndrome: a distinct disease entity. J Pediatr 2004;144:93–9.
2. Engelhardt KR, McGhee S, Winkler S, et al. Large deletions and point mutations involving the dedicator of cytokinesis 8 (DOCK8) in the autosomal-recessive form of hyper-IgE syndrome. J Allergy Clin Immunol 2009;124:1289–302.e4.

3. Zhang Q, Davis JC, Lamborn IT, et al. Combined immunodeficiency associated with DOCK8 mutations. N Engl J Med 2009;361:2046–55.

4. Dobbs K, Dominguez Conde C, Zhang SY, et al. Inherited DOCK2 deficiency in patients with early-onset invasive infections. N Engl J Med 2015;372: 2409–22.

5. Zhang Q, Davis JC, Dove CG, et al. Genetic, clinical, and laboratory markers for DOCK8 immunodeficiency syndrome. Dis Markers 2010;29:131–9.

6. Aydin SE, Kilic SS, Aytekin C, et al. DOCK8 deficiency: clinical and immunological phenotype and treatment options - a review of 136 patients. J Clin Immunol 2015;35:189–98.

7. Engelhardt KR, Gertz ME, Keles S, et al. The extended clinical phenotype of 64 patients with dedicator of cytokinesis 8 deficiency. J Allergy Clin Immunol 2015;136:402–12.

8. Chu EY, Freeman AF, Jing H, et al. Cutaneous manifestations of DOCK8 deficiency syndrome. Arch Dermatol 2012;148:79–84.

9. Al-Herz W, Ragupathy R, Massaad MJ, et al. Clinical, immunologic and genetic profiles of DOCK8-deficient patients in Kuwait. Clin Immunol 2012; 143:266–72.

10. Shah NN, Freeman AF, Parta M, et al. Haploidentical transplantation for DOCK8 deficiency. 57th Annual Meeting and Exposition of the American Society of Hematology. December 5-8, Orlando, FL, 2015.

11. Caracciolo S, Moratto D, Giacomelli M, et al. Expansion of CCR4+ activated T cells is associated with memory B cell reduction in DOCK8-deficient patients. Clin Immunol 2014;152:164–70.

12. Randall KL, Chan SS, Ma CS, et al. DOCK8 deficiency impairs CD8 T cell survival and function in humans and mice. J Exp Med 2011;208:2305–20.

13. Dasouki M, Okonkwo KC, Ray A, et al. Deficient T Cell Receptor Excision Circles (TRECs) in autosomal recessive hyper IgE syndrome caused by DOCK8 mutation: implications for pathogenesis and potential detection by newborn screening. Clin Immunol 2011;141:128–32.

14. Janssen E, Tsitsikov E, Al-Herz W, et al. Flow cytometry biomarkers distinguish DOCK8 deficiency from severe atopic dermatitis. Clin Immunol 2014;150: 220–4.

15. Boos AC, Hagl B, Schlesinger A, et al. Atopic dermatitis, STAT3- and DOCK8-hyper-IgE syndromes differ in IgE-based sensitization pattern. Allergy 2014;69:943–53.

16. Grimbacher B, Schaffer AA, Holland SM, et al. Genetic linkage of hyper-IgE syndrome to chromosome 4. Am J Hum Genet 1999;65:735–44.

17. Hagl B, Heinz V, Schlesinger A, et al. Key findings to expedite the diagnosis of hyper-IgE syndromes in infants and young children. Pediatr Allergy Immunol 2016;27(2):177–84.

18. Moulding DA, Record J, Malinova D, et al. Actin cytoskeletal defects in immunodeficiency. Immunol Rev 2013;256:282–99.

19. Zhang Y, Yu X, Ichikawa M, et al. Autosomal recessive phosphoglucomutase 3 (PGM3) mutations link glycosylation defects to atopy, immune deficiency, autoimmunity, and neurocognitive impairment. J Allergy Clin Immunol 2014;133:1400–9, 1409.e1-5.

20. Chinn IK, Shearer WT. Severe combined immunodeficiency disorders. Immunol Allergy Clin N Am 2015; 35:671–94.

21. Halacli SO, Ayvaz DC, Sun-Tan C, et al. STK4 (MST1) deficiency in two siblings with autoimmune cytopenias: a novel mutation. Clin Immunol 2015; 161:316–23.

22. Kreins AY, Ciancanelli MJ, Okada S, et al. Human TYK2 deficiency: mycobacterial and viral infections without hyper-IgE syndrome. J Exp Med 2015;212: 1641–62.

23. Ruusala A, Aspenstrom P. Isolation and characterisation of DOCK8, a member of the DOCK180-related regulators of cell morphology. FEBS Lett 2004;572:159–66.

24. Cote JF, Vuori K. Identification of an evolutionarily conserved superfamily of DOCK180-related proteins with guanine nucleotide exchange activity. J Cell Sci 2002;115:4901–13.

25. Su HC. Dedicator of cytokinesis 8 (DOCK8) deficiency. Curr Opin Allergy Clin Immunol 2010;10: 515–20.

26. Harada Y, Tanaka Y, Terasawa M, et al. DOCK8 is a Cdc42 activator critical for interstitial dendritic cell migration during immune responses. Blood 2012; 119:4451–61.

27. Al-Zahrani D, Raddadi A, Massaad M, et al. Successful interferon-alpha 2b therapy for unremitting warts in a patient with DOCK8 deficiency. Clin Immunol 2014;153:104–8.

28. Keles S, Jabara HH, Reisli I, et al. Plasmacytoid dendritic cell depletion in DOCK8 deficiency: rescue of severe herpetic infections with IFN-alpha 2b therapy. J Allergy Clin Immunol 2014;133:1753–5.e3.

29. Randall KL, Lambe T, Johnson AL, et al. Dock8 mutations cripple B cell immunological synapses, germinal centers and long-lived antibody production. Nat Immunol 2009;10:1283–91.

30. Jabara HH, McDonald DR, Janssen E, et al. DOCK8 functions as an adaptor that links TLR-MyD88 signaling to B cell activation. Nat Immunol 2012; 13:612–20.

31. Flesch IE, Randall KL, Hollett NA, et al. Delayed control of herpes simplex virus infection and impaired CD4(+) T-cell migration to the skin in mouse models of DOCK8 deficiency. Immunol Cell Biol 2015;93: 517–21.

32. Lambe T, Crawford G, Johnson AL, et al. DOCK8 is essential for T-cell survival and the maintenance of

CD8+ T-cell memory. Eur J Immunol 2011;41: 3423–35.

33. Ham H, Guerrier S, Kim J, et al. Dedicator of cytokinesis 8 interacts with talin and Wiskott-Aldrich syndrome protein to regulate NK cell cytotoxicity. J Immunol 2013;190:3661–9.

34. McGhee SA, Chatila TA. DOCK8 immune deficiency as a model for primary cytoskeletal dysfunction. Dis Markers 2010;29:151–6.

35. Mizesko MC, Banerjee PP, Monaco-Shawver L, et al. Defective actin accumulation impairs human natural killer cell function in patients with dedicator of cytokinesis 8 deficiency. J Allergy Clin Immunol 2013; 131:840–8.

36. Zhang Q, Dove CG, Hor JL, et al. DOCK8 regulates lymphocyte shape integrity for skin antiviral immunity. J Exp Med 2014;211:2549–66.

37. Crawford G, Enders A, Gileadi U, et al. DOCK8 is critical for the survival and function of NKT cells. Blood 2013;122:2052–61.

38. Sato M, Takahashi K, Nagayama K, et al. Identification of chromosome arm 9p as the most frequent target of homozygous deletions in lung cancer. Genes Chromosomes Cancer 2005;44:405–14.

39. Takahashi K, Kohno T, Ajima R, et al. Homozygous deletion and reduced expression of the DOCK8 gene in human lung cancer. Int J Oncol 2006;28: 321–8.

40. Takada H, Imoto I, Tsuda H, et al. Genomic loss and epigenetic silencing of very-low-density lipoprotein receptor involved in gastric carcinogenesis. Oncogene 2006;25:6554–62.

41. Heidenblad M, Schoenmakers EF, Jonson T, et al. Genome-wide array-based comparative genomic hybridization reveals multiple amplification targets and novel homozygous deletions in pancreatic carcinoma cell lines. Cancer Res 2004;64:3052–9.

42. Saelee P, Wongkham S, Puapairoj A, et al. Novel PNLIPRP3 and DOCK8 gene expression and prognostic implications of DNA loss on chromosome 10q25.3 in hepatocellular carcinoma. Asian Pac J Cancer Prev 2009;10:501–6.

43. Idbaih A, Carvalho Silva R, Criniere E, et al. Genomic changes in progression of low-grade gliomas. J Neurooncol 2008;90:133–40.

44. Marescalco MS, Capizzi C, Condorelli DF, et al. Genome-wide analysis of recurrent copy-number alterations and copy-neutral loss of heterozygosity in head and neck squamous cell carcinoma. J Oral Pathol Med 2014;43:20–7.

45. Ogawa R, Ishiguro H, Kuwabara Y, et al. Identification of candidate genes involved in the radiosensitivity of esophageal cancer cells by microarray analysis. Dis Esophagus 2008;21:288–97.

46. Wang SJ, Cui HY, Liu YM, et al. CD147 promotes Src-dependent activation of Rac1 signaling through STAT3/DOCK8 during the motility of hepatocellular carcinoma cells. Oncotarget 2015;6:243–57.

47. McDonald DR, Massaad MJ, Johnston A, et al. Successful engraftment of donor marrow after allogeneic hematopoietic cell transplantation in autosomal-recessive hyper-IgE syndrome caused by dedicator of cytokinesis 8 deficiency. J Allergy Clin Immunol 2010;126:1304–5.e3.

48. Pai SY, de Boer H, Massaad MJ, et al. Flow cytometry diagnosis of dedicator of cytokinesis 8 (DOCK8) deficiency. J Allergy Clin Immunol 2014;134:221–3.

49. Bittner TC, Pannicke U, Renner ED, et al. Successful long-term correction of autosomal recessive hyper-IgE syndrome due to DOCK8 deficiency by hematopoietic stem cell transplantation. Klin Padiatr 2010; 222:351–5.

50. Gatz SA, Benninghoff U, Schutz C, et al. Curative treatment of autosomal-recessive hyper-IgE syndrome by hematopoietic cell transplantation. Bone Marrow Transplant 2011;46:552–6.

51. Metin A, Tavil B, Azik F, et al. Successful bone marrow transplantation for DOCK8 deficient hyper IgE syndrome. Pediatr Transplant 2012;16:398–9.

52. Boztug H, Karitnig-Weiss C, Ausserer B, et al. Clinical and immunological correction of DOCK8 deficiency by allogeneic hematopoietic stem cell transplantation following a reduced toxicity conditioning regimen. Pediatr Hematol Oncol 2012;29: 585–94.

53. Ghosh S, Schuster FR, Fuchs I, et al. Treosulfan-based conditioning in DOCK8 deficiency: complete lympho-hematopoietic reconstitution with minimal toxicity. Clin Immunol 2012;145:259–61.

54. Cuellar-Rodriguez J, Freeman AF, Grossman J, et al. Matched related and unrelated donor hematopoietic stem cell transplantation for DOCK8 deficiency. Biol Blood Marrow Transplant 2015;21:1037–45.

55. Purcell C, Cant A, Irvine AD. DOCK8 primary immunodeficiency syndrome. Lancet 2015;386:982.

56. Ghosh S, Schuster FR, Adams O, et al. Haploidentical stem cell transplantation in DOCK8 deficiency: successful control of pre-existing severe viremia with a TCRass/CD19-depleted graft and antiviral treatment. Clin Immunol 2014;152:111–4.

57. Barlogis V, Galambrun C, Chambost H, et al. Successful allogeneic hematopoietic stem cell transplantation for DOCK8 deficiency. J Allergy Clin Immunol 2011;128:420–2.e2.

58. Jing H, Zhang Q, Zhang Y, et al. Somatic reversion in dedicator of cytokinesis 8 immunodeficiency modulates disease phenotype. J Allergy Clin Immunol 2014;133:1667–75.

Dermatologic Manifestations of Monogenic Autoinflammatory Diseases

Kyawt Win Shwin, MD[a,b], Chyi-Chia Richard Lee, MD, PhD[c], Raphaela Goldbach-Mansky, MD, MHS[d,*]

KEYWORDS

- Autoinflammatory disorders • IL-1 • Type I interferon • Immune dysregulation
- Neutrophilic dermatoses • urticaria • Panniculitis

KEY POINTS

- Monogenic autoinflammatory disorders are hyperinflammatory conditions caused by single-gene mutations in innate immune regulatory pathways. They often present in infancy or early childhood; some can mimic infection or sepsis.
- Recognizing the clinical and histologic features is essential in initiating genetic testing, appropriate referral to make an early diagnosis, and to begin aggressive treatment to prevent organ damage and life-threatening consequences.
- Patients with interleukin (IL)-1–mediated disorders present with neutrophilic urticaria, pustulosis, and migratory rash, whereas interferon (IFN)-mediated disorders may present with panniculitis, livedo reticularis, or vasculitis.
- Anti–IL-1 therapy is the standard of care in treating the cryopyrinopathies (cryopyrin-associated periodic syndrome), and deficiency of IL-1 receptor antagonist and other IL-1–mediated conditions, including familial Mediterranean fever, hyperimmunoglobulinemia D syndrome, and tumor necrosis factor receptor–associated periodic syndrome.
- Discoveries of the genetic cause of novel autoinflammatory diseases suggest a role for type I IFN, IL-17, and IL-18; several have uncovered novel targets for therapeutic intervention.

INTRODUCTION

Autoinflammatory disorders are immune-dysregulatory conditions characterized by early onset, sterile systemic inflammatory episodes that include fever, rashes, joint pain, and features of disease-specific organ inflammation.[1] The term autoinflammatory was proposed by Daniel Kastner in 1999 after the discovery of the genetic causes of the familial Mediterranean

Disclosure: R. Goldbach-Mansky received study support from SOBI, Novartis, Regeneron and Eli Lilly. The authors are supported by the Intramural Research Program of the NIH, NIAID, NIAMS, and NCI.

[a] Translational Autoinflammatory Disease Studies, Rheumatology Fellowship Program, National Institutes of Arthritis and Musculoskeletal and Skin Diseases (NIAMS), National Institutes of Health (NIH), Building 10, Room 6D-52, 10 Center Drive, Bethesda, MD 20892, USA; [b] Division of Rheumatic Diseases, UT Southwestern Medical Center, Dallas VA Medical Center, North Texas Health Care System, 4500 S. Lancaster Road, Dallas, TX 75216, USA; [c] Dermatopathology Section, Laboratory of Pathology, Center for Cancer Research (CCR), National Cancer Institute (NCI), National Institutes of Health (NIH), Building 10, Room 2S235J, 9000 Rockville Pike, Bethesda, MD 20892, USA; [d] Translational Autoinflammatory Disease Studies, National Institute of Allergy and Infectious Diseases (NIAID), National Institutes of Health (NIH), Building 10, Room 6D-47B, 10 Center Drive, Bethesda, MD 20892, USA

* Corresponding author.

E-mail address: goldbacr@mail.nih.gov

derm.theclinics.com

fever (FMF)[2,3] and of the tumor necrosis factor (TNF) receptor–associated periodic syndrome (TRAPS).[4]

Over the last 15 years the discovery of the genetic causes for several autoinflammatory diseases revealed gain-of-function (GOF) mutations in intracellular innate immune sensors (**Fig. 1**), including the interleukin (IL)-1 and IL-18 activating inflammasomes *MEFV*/pyrin, *NLRP3*/cryopyrin, and nod-like receptor (NLR) family CARD domain-containing protein 4 (*NLRC4*); *NLRC4* also leads to high IL-18 serum levels. Mutations in the NOD-like receptor NOD2/caspase recruitment domain family, member 15 (CARD15) cause constitutive nuclear factor kappa B (NF-κB) activation; and more recently mutations in the viral RIG-I–like receptors, *IFIH1/MDA-5*[5] and DDX58, or the adaptor molecule *TMEM173/STING*[6] encoding the stimulator of interferon genes (STING), are all linked to type I interferon (IFN) production and cause autoinflammatory phenotypes. Furthermore, loss-of-function (LOF) mutations in genes (ie, many of the enzymes) involved in protein or nucleic acid metabolism, cell transport, and other cellular homeostatic functions can lead to the accumulation of intracellular danger signals, which can trigger innate immune sensors and activate proinflammatory pathways (see **Fig. 1**). The

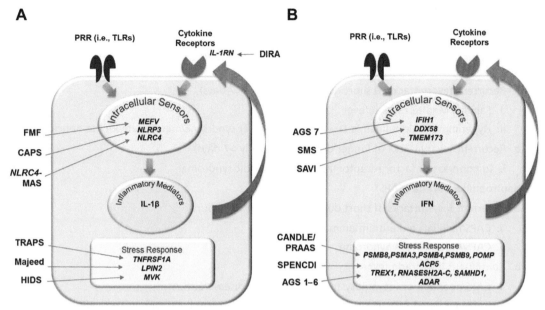

Fig. 1. IL-1-mediated and IFN Type I –mediated autoinflammatory diseases (AIDs) and their genetic causes. (*A*) IL-1-mediated. (*B*) Type I IFN-mediated. AGS 1-6, Aicardi–Goutières syndrome 1-6; AGS 7, Aicardi–Goutières syndrome 7; CANDLE, chronic atypical neutrophilic dermatosis with lipodystrophy and elevated temperature; CAPS, cryopyrin-associated periodic syndrome (including the severity specrtum of FCAS, familial cold autoinflammatory syndrome; MWS, muckle–wells syndrome; NOMID, neonatal-onset multisystem inflammatory disease); DIRA, deficiency of interleukin-1 receptor antagonist; FMF, familial Mediterranean fever; MKD, mevalonate kinase deficiency or HIDS, hyperimmunoglobulinemia D and periodic fever syndrome; *NLRC4*-MAS, NLRC4-associated macrophage activation syndrome which is also IL-18 mediated; PRAAS, proteasome-associated autoinflammatory syndrome; PRR, Pattern recognition receptor; SAVI, STING-associated vasculopathy with onset in infancy; SMS, Singleton–Merten syndrome; SPENCDI, Spodyloenchondrodysplasia with immune dysregulation; TLRs, toll-like receptors; TRAPS, TNF receptor-associated periodic syndrome. (*Adapted from* Jesus AA, Canna SW, Liu Y, et al. Molecular mechanisms in autoinflammatory diseases: disorders of amplified danger sensing. Annu Rev Immunol 2015;33:823–74. PMID: 25706096; with permission.)

increased and often constitutive release of the proinflammatory cytokines IL-1β, type I IFN, and TNF leads to autocrine cytokine amplification loops and these have become the targets for therapies. Although targeting IL-1 blockade therapeutically has become the treatment of choice for the IL-1–mediated diseases, targeting TNF is used empirically in some conditions and drugs targeting type I IFN or IL-18 are currently being used as compassionate use therapies.

Many monogenic autoinflammatory disorders present with characteristic skin rashes and cutaneous neutrophilic inflammation and patients are often referred to dermatologists for evaluation of the dermatologic findings and skin biopsies. It is therefore important for dermatologists to be familiar with these conditions because specific treatments can be life changing for many patients. This article presents groupings of autoinflammatory diseases based on dermatologic manifestations and fever patterns that allow a preliminary diagnosis based on systemic and dermatologic manifestations before

genetic testing results become available (**Box 1, Table 1**).

INTERLEUKIN-1–MEDIATED AUTOINFLAMMATORY DISEASES
Nonspecific Maculopapular Rashes with Recurrent Episodic Fever and Abdominal Pain Hereditary Periodic Fever Syndromes

The hereditary fever syndromes are characterized by episodic and periodic high fever attacks that are accompanied by abdominal and/or chest pain followed by periods of remission or reduced inflammation. They include FMF, hyperimmunoglobulinemia D and periodic fever syndrome (HIDS), and TRAPS.

Familial Mediterranean fever
FMF is an early onset autosomal recessive disorder caused by GOF mutation in the *MEFV* gene, which encodes pyrin, which leads to unregulated release of proinflammatory cytokines, such as IL-1β, and uncontrolled inflammation. Autosomal

Box 1
Dermatologic manifestations of monogenic autoinflammatory diseases

1. Nonspecific maculopapular rashes with recurrent episodic fever and abdominal pain (hereditary periodic fever syndrome)
   a. Recurrent fever attacks of short duration (typically ≤7 days)
      i. Familial Mediterranean fever
      ii. Hyperimmunoglobulinemia D with periodic fever syndrome/mevalonate kinase deficiency
   b. Recurrent fever attacks of longer duration (typically >7 days)
      i. Tumor necrosis factor receptor–associated periodic syndrome
2. Neutrophilic urticaria (CAPS)
   a. Recurrent fever attacks of short duration (typically <24 hours)
      i. CAPS/familial cold autoinflammatory syndrome
      ii. CAPS/Muckle-Wells Syndrome
   b. Continuous low-grade fever
      i. CAPS/neonatal-onset multisystem inflammatory disease/CINCA
      ii. IL-18–mediated AID and IL-1–mediated AID: NLRC4-related macrophage activation syndrome
3. Pustular skin rashes and episodic fevers
   a. IL-1–mediated pyogenic disorders with sterile osteomyelitis
      i. Deficiency of IL-1 receptor antagonist
      ii. Majeed syndrome
   b. Partially IL-1–mediated pyogenic disorders
      i. Pyogenic sterile arthritis, pyoderma gangrenosum, and acne syndrome
      ii. Haploinsufficiency of A20 (monogenic form of Behçet disease)
   c. Pyogenic disorders caused by non–IL-1 cytokine dysregulation
      i. Deficiency of IL-36 receptor antagonist
      ii. CARD14-mediated psoriasis (monogenic form of psoriasis)
      iii. Early-onset inflammatory bowel disease
4. Vasculopathy and panniculitis/lipoatrophy syndromes
   a. Chronic atypical neutrophilic dermatitis with lipodystrophy and elevated temperature syndrome or proteasome-associated autoinflammatory syndrome
5. Vasculopathy and/or vasculitis with livedo reticularis syndromes
   a. Without significant CNS disease
      i. STING-associated vasculopathy with onset in infancy
   b. With severe CNS disease
      i. Aicardi-Goutières syndrome
      ii. Deficiency of adenosine deaminase 2
      iii. Spondyloenchondrodysplasia with immune dysregulation
6. Autoinflammatory disorders with granulomatous skin diseases
   a. Without significant immunodeficiency
      i. Blau syndrome (pediatric granulomatous arthritis, pediatric granulomatous arthritis)
   b. With variable features of immunodeficiency and significant CNS disease
      i. PLCγ2-associated antibody deficiency and immune dysregulation: cold-induced urticaria and/or granulomatous rash

7. Other autoinflammatory syndromes

 a. *LACC1*-mediated monogenic Still disease

Abbreviations: AID, autoinflammatory disorder; CAPS, cryopyrin-associated periodic syndromes; CINCA, chronic infantile neurological cutaneous and articular syndrome; CNS, central nervous system.

dominant forms of the disease exist. The inflammatory attacks typically last for 3 to 7 days and recur every 4 to 6 weeks, and are accompanied by severe abdominal pain and to a lesser degree chest pain caused by sterile serositis. Debilitating myalgia with normal creatine kinase (CK) levels and sometimes synovitis is also seen. During the attacks, inflammatory markers, erythrocyte sedimentation rate (ESR), and C- reactive protein (CRP) level are highly increased and may normalize between attacks. Patients from Armenia, Turkey, and Arabian countries with a long-standing history of FMF are at high risk of developing AA amyloidosis leading to renal failure.

Cutaneous manifestations The prevalence of pathognomonic erysipelaslike erythema (**Fig. 2**A) varies widely among different populations (21% and 46% in Turks and Jews, but 3% and 8% in Arabs and Armenians[7]), and it occurs on the distal extremities. The lesions present as tender, warm, swollen, and erythematous plaques that are triggered by prolonged walking and subside within 24 to 48 hours. Other rarer eruptions include scattered nonspecific purpuric papules[8]; nodules have also been reported in children with FMF.[9]

Dermatopathology Biopsies of cutaneous eruptions reveal dermal edema with a perivascular and interstitial dermal infiltrate composed of neutrophils and lymphocytes (**Fig. 2**B). Mild hyperkeratosis and acanthosis can be seen in the epidermis.[10,11]

Treatment Colchicine is used as a first-line therapy to treat attacks and to prevent amyloidosis. IL-1 inhibition is effective but is mainly used in colchicine-refractory cases.

Hyperimmunoglobulinemia D and periodic fever syndrome
HIDS is an autosomal recessive disorder caused by LOF mutations in the gene *MVK* encoding for mevalonate kinase, an enzyme involved in

Table 1
Clinical features of interleukin-1–mediated versus interferon-mediated autoinflammatory disorders

IL-1-mediated AIDs	IFN-mediated AIDs
Systemic	
CRP closely correlates with disease activity	CRP level only increased in severe disease
Granulocytosis with flares	Lymphopenia, leukopenia with flares
CNS	
Aseptic neutrophilic meningitis	Mild lymphocytic meningitis
Arachnoid adhesions (severe disease)	Basal ganglion calcifications, CNS vasculopathy, white matter disease
Other Organ Involvements	
Skin, vessels: neutrophilic dermatitis (urticarialike with mature neutrophilic infiltrates)	Panniculitis (immature neutrophils), lipoatrophy, vasculitis (chilblainlike lesions), microthrombotic disease
Lung/heart: serositis, pericarditis	Pulmonary fibrosis/interstitial lung disease, HTN, Pulmonary HTN
MSK: osteomyelitis, bony overgrowth, fasciitis	Myositis
ENT: hearing loss (inflammatory)	NA
Eyes: conjunctivitis, anterior uveitis	Glaucoma, episcleritis
Serology: 40% lupus anticoagulant positive	Some with increased autoantibodies

Abbreviations: AIDs, autoinflammatory disorders; CNS, central nervous system; CRP, C-reactive protein; ENT, ear, nose, throat; HTN, hypertension; MSK, musculoskeletal manifestations; NA, not applicable.
 Adapted from Canna SW, Goldbach-Mansky R. New monogenic autoinflammatory diseases—a clinical overview. Semin Immunopathol 2015;37(4):387–94; with permission.

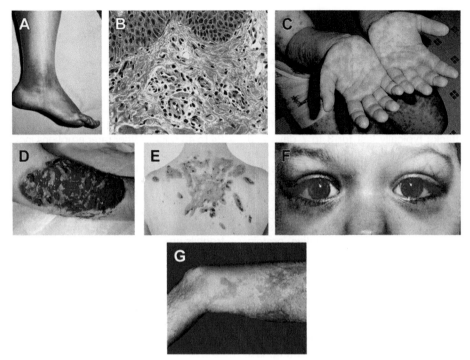

Fig. 2. (*A*) FMF: well-demarcated, swollen, bright erythematous erysipelaslike skin eruption on right ankle. (*B*) Histology of skin biopsy of affected skin from a patient with FMF showed a mild perivascular chronic inflammatory infiltrate in dermis. (*C*) HIDS: diffuse erythematous macules and papules over both palms, arms, legs, and trunk (not shown) during fever attack. (*D*). Pyoderma gangrenosum in pyogenic sterile arthritis, pyoderma gangrenosum and acne (PAPA): a large, ulcerated lesion with granulation tissue and purulent exudate at the ulcer base. (*E*) PAPA: severe cystic acnes with hypertrophic scars. (*F*) TRAPS: periorbital edema. (*G*) Erythematous patch on the leg of a patient with TRAPS.

cholesterol synthesis.[12] Patients with HIDS present with fever attacks that last from 3 to 7 days; tender cervical lymphadenopathy, arthralgia, nonerosive arthritis, and commonly with abdominal pain; and vomiting and diarrhea. Hepatomegaly and splenomegaly are seen in a quarter to a third of patients and serositis is less frequent. During attacks, patients have very high levels of inflammatory markers, ESR, CRP levels, and leukocytosis, which may continue to be increased between attacks. High serum immunoglobulin (Ig) D level may assist in making the diagnosis but this can be normal in a quarter of all patients. The frequency of the attacks often decreases with increasing age. Only about 3% of patients with long-standing disease develop type AA amyloidosis. Other rare complications include abdominal adhesions from repeated peritonitis and joint contractures.

Cutaneous manifestations Skin lesions vary with fever attacks and are seen in more than two-thirds of patients with HIDS. They include maculopapular, morbilliform, nodular, and purpuric rashes (**Fig. 2**C). Behçet-like aphthae with or without genital ulcerations develop in almost 50% of these patients.[13,14]

Dermatopathology Biopsies of affected skin show endothelial cell swelling, fibrinoid necrosis of vessel walls, and a perivascular neutrophilic and lymphocytic infiltrate. Slight leukocytoclasia and features of leukocytoclastic vasculitis can be seen. By direct immunofluorescence, perivascular deposits of IgD and C3 in a granular staining pattern are found in skin samples from some patients.[15]

Treatment Nonsteroidal antiinflammatory drugs (NSAIDs), prednisone, and IL-1 blockade have been the treatments of choice. TNF inhibition (etanercept) can be effective in some patients in reducing the severity of disease flares, but colchicine, thalidomide, and cyclosporine are ineffective.[16]

Tumor necrosis factor receptor–associated periodic syndrome
TNF receptor–associated periodic syndrome (TRAPS) is a dominantly inherited disorder

caused by LOF mutations in the *TNFRSF1A* gene encoding TNF-alpha receptor 1 that results in retention of mutant TNF receptor in the Golgi apparatus and an inflammatory reaction that is complex and involves increased TNF and IL-1 production and signaling.[17,18] Patients present with recurrent fever and abdominal pain, pleurisy, and joint pain that can resemble FMF attacks. However, the attacks are longer and can last from 1 to several weeks and recur every 4 to 6 weeks; the intervals between attacks can be greater. Clinical manifestations include conjunctivitis and periorbital edema (**Fig. 2**F), and rarely uveitis and iritis. Acute phase reactants such as ESR, CRP, haptoglobin, fibrinogen, and ferritin levels can be increased during inflammatory attacks in all hereditary fever syndromes. Autoantibodies to antinuclear antibody (ANA), RF, or antineutrophil cytoplasmic antibody (ANCA) are not usually found. Systemic AA amyloidosis with development of nephrotic syndrome and renal failure is a very severe complication of TRAPS.

Cutaneous manifestations Patients with TRAPS often complain of focal migratory myalgia that underlies centrifugal, migratory, tender, well-demarcated, blanchable, erythematous plaques, often on the lower legs (**Fig. 2**G). The lesions develop during early childhood as warm, urticarial, erythematous macules and plaques.

Dermatopathology On histopathology, a mild perivascular lymphocytic infiltrate is often present in the edematous areas of the papillary dermis. Slight perivascular C3 and C4 deposition in the dermis has been described.[19] A fascial biopsy shows no histologic evidence of myositis but a dense inflammatory infiltrate surrounding connective tissue, including focal panniculitis, fasciitis, and perivascular chronic inflammation.[20]

Treatment Corticosteroids and anti-TNF agents suppress the attacks and control the disease activity and severity. IL-1 blockade shows satisfactory responses and has become the agent of choice in many instances and is beneficial in patients with a high risk for the development of amyloidosis.[16,21,22] Colchicine is not effective in patients with TRAPS.

Neutrophilic Urticaria (the Cryopyrin-Associated Periodic Syndrome)

The 3 conditions, familial cold autoinflammatory syndrome (FCAS), Muckle-Wells syndrome (MWS), and neonatal-onset multisystem inflammatory disease (NOMID), also known as chronic infantile, neurologic, cutaneous, and articular (CINCA), listed in increasing disease severity, are referred to as cryopyrin-associated periodic syndrome (CAPS).

Autosomal dominant GOF mutations in *NLRP3* lead to unchecked inflammasome activation in patients with CAPS.[23,24] The hallmarks of all CAPS include a nonpruritic neutrophilic urticaria on the trunk, extremities, and face associated with low-grade fevers, conjunctivitis, arthralgia, and increased acute phase reactant levels during active disease. Inflammatory attacks in NOMID may mimic neonatal sepsis early in life. Ocular manifestations are not always present in FCAS attacks, but conjunctivitis, episcleritis, and uveitis are seen in patients with MWS and NOMID. Patients with MWS often develop sensorineural hearing loss in the second and third decades of life. NOMID is the most severe form of CAPS, with hearing loss developing in the first decade of life. Patients present with aseptic meningitis with neutrophilic pleocytosis; hydrocephalus and cognitive impairment can develop in patients with NOMID who do not receive early appropriate treatment.

Cutaneous manifestations
In FCAS, low ambient temperatures trigger inflammatory attacks, which resolve within a few hours, whereas urticaria (**Fig. 3**A) may develop at birth or within hours of birth in patients with MWS and NOMID and is typically not induced by cold. The skin lesions in patients with FCAS and patients with the other CAPS are intermittent, migratory, and nonscarring; the ice cube test is negative.

Dermatopathology
On histology, the epidermis is unaffected in CAPS. Mild edema of the papillary dermis and dilatation of superficial dermal capillaries can be seen. Predominantly neutrophilic, perieccrine, and perivascular infiltrates are noted throughout the dermis (**Fig. 3**B–D); there is no evidence of vasculopathy or vasculitis. Histologic findings of neutrophilic infiltrates in lesional skin differ from classic urticaria, in which lymphocytes and eosinophils are the predominant inflammatory cells.

Treatment
IL-1 inhibition with anakinra, a recombinant human IL-1 receptor antagonist (US Food and Drug Administration [FDA] approved for NOMID) and long-acting blockers (rilonacept and canakinumab, FDA approved for FCAS and MWS) are standard of care. Treatment results in rapid improvement of inflammatory symptoms. Early

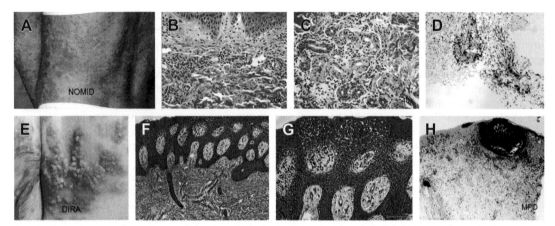

Fig. 3. Cutaneous manifestations and dermatopathology of NOMID (*A–D*) and deficiency of interleukin 1 receptor antagonist (DIRA) (*E–H*). (*A*) Diffuse erythematous papules and plaques of urticarial rash of a patient with NOMID. (*B*) Skin biopsy section from a patient with NOMID showing perivascular neutrophilic infiltrates in the superficial dermis and surrounding sweat glands (*C*). (*D*) Myeloperoxidase-positive (MPO+; mature neutrophils) cellular inflammatory infiltrates (*dark brown*) in dermis. (*E*) Erythematous patch with papules, vesicles, and pustules in a patient with DIRA. (*F, G*). Intracorneal and intraepidermal neutrophilic microabscesses in the affected skin of a patient with DIRA. (*H*) Dense MPO+ cells (*dark brown*) within an intraepidermal abscess.

initiation of treatment is crucial to prevent disease progression and organ damage.[16]

Autoinflammatory Disease Mediated by Interleukin-18/Interleukin-1

NLRC4-related macrophage activation syndrome

NLRC4-related macrophage activation syndrome (MAS) is caused by GOF mutations in *NLRC4*, which encodes a protein that nucleates the *NLRC4* inflammasome. Disease-causing mutations lead to early onset fever flares and predispose to the development of MAS.[25,26] In the perinatal period early onset enterocolitis with periodic fevers can be seen. Characteristic features of MAS flares are caused by uncontrolled macrophage activation and include persistent fever, extreme hyperferritinemia, transaminitis, variable lymphadenopathy and hepatosplenomegaly, increased CRP level, initially high then decreasing ESR, and rapidly progressing pancytopenia that are partially caused by macrophage hemophagocytosis. As MAS progresses, hypertriglyceridemia, serum fibrinogen level, and D-dimer level increase are associated with multiorgan failure. The mortality of untreated MAS is high.

Unlike patients with CAPS and other autoinflammatory diseases, patients with *NLRC4* mutations have extremely high serum IL-18 levels, comparable with levels seen in other conditions that are prone to the development of MAS, such as systemic juvenile idiopathic arthritis and some adult forms of Still disease.[25,27,28] Patients can present with variable severity of gastrointestinal inflammation in early infancy.

Cutaneous manifestations Cutaneous manifestations of NLRC4-MAS can vary and include an evanescent rash with dermographism and linear erythemalike lesions,[25,26] whereas other patients present with an urticarialike rash and fever flares similar to those seen in patients with CAPS with *NLRP3* mutations.[29]

Dermatopathology Histology of skin biopsies is not currently available. Histologic examination of a duodenal mucosal biopsy shows mixed inflammatory infiltrate in the lamina propria and mild villous blunting.[25]

Treatment Corticosteroids and IL-1 blockade can alleviate inflammatory flares. However, high serum IL-18 levels may persist even after IL-1 inhibition therapy.

Pustular Skin Rashes and Episodic Fevers

The conditions listed here are a pathogenically heterogeneous group of autoinflammatory disorders, all of which present with pustulosis.

Interleukin-1–mediated pyogenic disorders with sterile osteomyelitis

Deficiency of interleukin-1 receptor antagonist Deficiency of IL-1 receptor antagonist (DIRA) is a severe recessive disorder caused by LOF mutations in *IL1RN*, which encodes the IL-1 receptor antagonist.[30–32] Patients present with highly increased levels of acute phase reactants, multifocal periosteitis, bony overgrowth, and sterile painful osteomyelitis. Lesions involve the long bones, frequently the ribs, vertebra, and skull. Odontoid involvement can lead to atlantoaxial subluxation.

Cutaneous manifestations DIRA is characterized by neonatal-onset diffuse pustular dermatitis (**Fig. 3E**) that can appear in crops limited to 1 area or be generalized.

Dermatopathology Biopsies of skin lesions of patients with DIRA show dense myeloperoxidase-positive (MPO+) neutrophilic infiltrates in the epidermis and superficial dermis (**Fig. 3F–H**), formation of pustules around the hair shaft, acanthosis, and hyperkeratosis. Deep connective tissue may show evidence of vasculitis and perivascular neutrophilic infiltration.[30]

Treatment Antiinflammatory and replacement therapy with recombinant IL-1 receptor antagonist, anakinra is the treatment of choice and leads to complete remission.[30–32]

Majeed syndrome Majeed syndrome is caused by recessive LOF mutations in the *LPIN2* gene, which encodes a phosphatase, lipin2, which plays a nonredundant role in phospholipid processing in monocytes and macrophages and in innate immune responses. Patients with Majeed syndrome present with perinatal-onset recurrent osteitis and multifocal sterile osteomyelitis. Patients may present with mild or transfusion-dependent congenital hypochromic microcytic anemia.

Cutaneous manifestations Skin eruptions are described as Sweet syndrome–like lesions and other forms of neutrophilic dermatoses, including pustulosis and severe psoriasis.[33] Skin lesions can be itchy with serosanguinous discharge.[34]

Dermatopathology Lesional skin biopsies show dermal neutrophilic infiltrate with edema of the upper dermis without histologic evidence of vasculitis.

Treatment IL-1 blockade is highly efficacious with dramatic improvement of inflammatory symptoms.[30–32,35–37]

Partially interleukin-1–mediated pyogenic disorders
Pyogenic sterile arthritis, pyoderma gangrenosum, and acne Pyogenic sterile arthritis, pyoderma gangrenosum, and acne (PAPA) syndrome is dominantly inherited and is caused by mutations in the *PSTPIP1* gene.[38] Arthritis may start in the first decade of life and can be progressively destructive. Increased levels of acute phase reactants are seen during disease flares but can be persistently high in patients with severe chronic and recalcitrant disease.

Cutaneous manifestations Skin eruptions can be triggered by minor trauma and usually begin as violaceous nodules on extremities or the face and result in chronic, poor-healing ulcers with undermined borders; severe cystic acnes may heal with scars (**Fig. 2D, E**).

Dermatopathology Histologic findings include inflammatory infiltrates composed predominantly of neutrophils in the dermis and superficial ulcerations.

Treatment The disease responds partially to systemic glucocorticoids. The pyogenic arthritis is usually responsive to IL-1 inhibition. However, patients with refractory skin lesions may need treatment with TNF-blocking agents (infliximab, adalimumab, etanercept) to obtain control of their skin disease. Optimal treatment still needs to be defined.

Haploinsufficiency of A20 Haploinsufficiency of A20 (HA20) is caused by autosomal dominant LOF mutations in *TNFAIP3*, leading to a ubiquitinylation defect that results in impaired regulatory function of A20 and upregulation of the NF-κB signaling pathway and multiorgan inflammation.[39] The condition is indistinguishable from the not genetically defined Behçet disease, and can be considered to be a monogenic form of Behçet disease. Symptoms start in early childhood or in adolescence. *TNFAIP3* gene polymorphisms have been associated with the prevalence of Behçet disease in the Chinese Han population.[40] Clinical features of HA20 include asymmetrical nondeforming polyarthritis of small and large joints, uveitis, retinal vasculitis, gastrointestinal manifestations such as colitis, diffuse ulcers in the oropharynx and colon, ulcers in the terminal ileum, and rarely central nervous system (CNS) vasculitis. Autoantibodies to ANA, ribonucleoprotein (RNP), double-stranded DNA (dsDNA), and lupus anticoagulant can be found.

Cutaneous manifestations Patients with HA20 present with oral and genital ulcers, and skin eruptions described in the not genetically defined Behçet disease, including papules, folliculitis, erythema nodosum–like lesions, and pathergy.

Dermatopathology Histologic findings for patients with HA20 have not been reported, but the spectrum of clinical lesions is similar to what is reported in patients with not yet genetically defined

Behçet disease and includes folliculitis and erythema nodosum–like lesions. In Behçet disease, features of neutrophilic vasculitis and the deposition of fibrinoid material within the vessel walls of arterioles and venules were seen in more than 40% of biopsied samples from patients[41] but it is unknown whether this is also a common feature in patients with HA20 Behçet.

Treatment Patients with HA20 respond to colchicine and TNF blockade with infliximab and anti–IL-1 therapy in refractory cases.[39]

Pyogenic disorders caused by non–interleukin-1 cytokine dysregulation

Deficiency of interleukin-36 receptor antagonist Deficiency of IL-36 receptor antagonist (DITRA) is an autosomal recessive disorder caused by homozygous or compound heterozygous LOF mutations in *IL36RN*, encoding IL-36 receptor antagonist (IL-36Ra), also known as IL-1F5. DITRA is characterized by recurrent episodes of high-grade fever, generalized pustular lesions, and with increased ESR, CRP level, and leukocytosis. IL-36Ra is an antagonist that binds to the IL-36 receptor (IL-36R) and downregulates IL-36alpha, IL-36beta, and IL-36gamma signaling (formerly named IL-1F6, IL-1F8, and IL-1F9). IL-36R is highly expressed on keratinocytes and hematopoietic cells and regulates the IL-23/IL-17/IL-22 pathway in the skin.[42] Disease flares are triggered by viral and bacterial infection, menstruation, and pregnancy. Other features include diarrhea with hypernatremia and dehydration followed by feeding difficulties and growth failure in young children. Gastric ulcers were also reported in a patient with DITRA.

Cutaneous manifestations Patients present with generalized scaly erythematous pustular eruptions, erythematous scaly plaques. The initial erythematous pustular lesions often precede desquamation of the leg and scalp. Psoriasis vulgaris, acral pustular lesions of the digits, nail dystrophy, impetigo herpetiformis, geographic tongue, and scrotal lesions have been described.[43]

Dermatopathology Skin biopsies show spongiosis with subcorneal pustules, acanthosis and parakeratosis, and a dense neutrophilic and lymphocytic infiltrate with CD3+ and CD8+ T cells. Dermal CD68+ and MPO+ cells are suggestive of tissue macrophages, and neutrophils are noted.

Treatment Optimal treatment of the disease is still challenging. Different therapeutic agents, such as topical steroids, oral glucocorticoids, retinoids, methotrexate, cyclosporine, adalimumab, etanercept, and infliximab, show variable individual responses. The use of anti–IL-17 and anti–IL-23 agents may be indicated but has not been reported so far.

CARD14-mediated psoriasis CARD14-mediated psoriasis (CAMPS) is dominantly inherited, by GOF mutations in *CARD14*, which is expressed in keratinocytes and endothelial cells but not in hematopoietic cells. The disease can present as a monogenic form of psoriasis vulgaris, or pustular psoriasis,[44] or as pityriasis rubra piliaris.[45] Variable disease expression is seen in affected family members. Mutant CARD14 leads to increased NF-κB translocation and increased production of chemokines by keratinocytes. It is hypothesized that tissue macrophages produce and secrete IL-23 and recruit and induce Th17 cell differentiation and the release of IL-17A and IL-17F, cytokines that are also produced by CD4+ and CD8+ T cells, γδ T cells, neutrophils, and mast cells. This process can induce a proinflammatory cytokine and chemokine milieu. Their target includes keratinocytes that become more activated[46,47] and fuel an abnormal amplification loop that further augments keratinocyte activation and inflammatory cell recruitment. In general, fever and other systemic manifestations are uncommon in the absence of superinfection of the skin in patients with CAMPS.

Cutaneous manifestations Patients with CAMPS present with a variable clinical severity spectrum from localized plaque and pustular psoriasis to the severe generalized manifestations of familial pityriasis rubra pilaris.

Dermatopathology Similarly, the histologic features vary and can range from those seen in plaque psoriasis, pustular psoriasis, and pityriasis rubra pilaris (PRP). The histologic features of PRP include acantholysis, hypergranulosis, follicular plugging, and the absence of psoriatic capillary alterations, granular layer diminution, and epidermal pustulation[48] may be considered to be at the severe end of the psoriasis/PRP severity spectrum.

Treatment The condition can be seen as a monogenic form of psoriasis and responds to the same treatments that are used for moderate to severe psoriasis, including methotrexate, cyclosporine, anti-TNF agents, IL-12/23p40 inhibitor (ustekinumab), IL-17A inhibitor (secukinumab), and other drugs targeting IL-17 and IL-23.[49]

Early onset of inflammatory bowel disease Early onset of inflammatory bowel disease (EO-IBD) is caused by autosomal recessive LOF mutations in either the *IL-10RA* or *IL-10RB* genes, encoding IL-1.[50] Patients with this mutation present with severe infantile inflammatory bowel disease, typically in the first 3 months of life, characterized by bloody diarrhea, colonic abscesses, perianal fistula, and oral ulcers. Other manifestations include chronic folliculitis, arthritis, fever, growth retardation, and delayed puberty. IL-10 inhibits proinflammatory cytokine release and action by blocking NF-κB–dependent signals and plays a critical role in maintaining mucosal homeostasis. Transmembrane IL-10R is a heterodimer and consists of the IL-10R-alpha and IL-10R-beta subunits that bind IL-10.[51,52] Colonoscopy shows moderate to severe colitis with an early cobblestone pattern, a mixed inflammatory infiltrate, and intermittent deep ulcerations and pseudopolyps.

Cutaneous manifestations Cutaneous manifestations include early onset recurrent folliculitis and enterocutaneous fistulas.

Treatment EO-IBD is a severe, therapy-refractory bowel disease. Patients often require surgical interventions, including partial or total colectomy.[50] Patients with EO-IBD, and particularly those with mutations in *IL-10R*, underwent hematopoietic stem cell transplant and achieved clinical remission.[50]

TYPE-1 INTERFERON–MEDIATED AUTOINFLAMMATORY DISEASES

Several conditions present with high type I IFN production and have been termed interferonopathies.[53] Mutations in viral sensors and enzymes regulating nucleic acid metabolism suggest that the accumulation of nucleotides may trigger viral sensors that drive the type I IFN response in some diseases. However, in other conditions, such as chronic atypical neutrophilic dermatitis with lipodystrophy and elevated temperature syndrome (CANDLE), the molecular pathways leading to the type I IFN response remain unknown. The conditions caused by nucleic acid dysregulation have a predilection for the development of severe neurologic and white matter disease when the disease presents in the first decade of life. The conditions presenting as autoinflammatory syndromes with high IFN scores can be grouped into 2 different categories depending on their cutaneous and vascular manifestations.

Vasculopathy and Panniculitis/Lipoatrophy Syndromes

Chronic atypical neutrophilic dermatitis with lipodystrophy and elevated temperature syndrome

CANDLE or proteasome-associated autoinflammatory syndromes (PRAAS), also known as Nakajo-Nishimura syndrome and joint contractures, muscle atrophy, microcytic anemia, and panniculitis-induced lipodystrophy (JMP), is caused by recessive mutations in *PSMB8*, and digenic mutations involving monoallelic changes in various combinations of *PSMB8*, *PSMB9*, *PSMA3*, and *PSMB4*. A monogenic autosomal dominant form with LOF mutations in proteasome maturation protein has been seen in 1 patient leading to impaired degradation of polyubiquitinylated proteins and type I IFN production.[54–59] Mechanisms of pathogenesis are still poorly understood. Clinical features include arthritis, joint contractures, fevers, myositis, hepatosplenomegaly, swelling of distal fingers, conjunctivitis, episcleritis, basal ganglia calcification, mild lymphocytic aseptic meningitis, metabolic syndrome, and later in life emaciation caused by lipoatrophy and muscle atrophy, and rarely cardiac arrhythmias and cardiomyopathy.[58,59] Transient thrombocytosis or thrombocytopenia, neutropenia, lymphopenia, hypertriglyceridemia, and increased acute phase reactant levels can be seen with flares.[60] Bone marrow suppression can develop over time with features of myelodysplasia.

Cutaneous manifestations CANDLE is characterized by early onset nodular erythematous eruptions (**Fig. 4**A) on trunk and extremities, and facial rashes that include red edematous, heliotropelike rashes and progressive facial lipoatrophy.

Dermatopathology Histologic findings include perivascular and interstitial mononuclear inflammatory infiltrates with karyorrhexis in the reticular dermis with extension into the subcutis (see **Fig. 4**B, C). Strong and diffuse MPO and chloroacetate esterase staining in skin biopsies support the presence of myeloid cells (see **Fig. 4**D, E). Intense positivity of CD68, and CD163, indicate the presence of histiocytes and macrophages. Moderate amounts of CD123+ cell infiltrates in the dermis represent the presence of plasmacytoid dendritic cells.[61]

Treatment Patients respond partially to steroids, but are refractory to NSAIDs, colchicine, dapsone, methotrexate, tacrolimus, azathioprine, TNF-blocking, IL-1–blocking, and IL-6–blocking agents.[60] Evidence of a strong IFN response gene signature in patients with CANDLE led to the compassionate use of the Janus kinase (JAK) inhibitor baricitinib, which blocks IFN receptor signaling through inhibition of JAK1/JAK2.[62]

Vasculopathy and/or Vasculitis with Livedo Reticularis Syndromes

Without significant central nervous system disease

Stimulator of interferon genes–associated vasculopathy with onset in infancy STING-associated vasculopathy with onset in infancy (SAVI) is caused by de novo GOF mutations in the gene *TMEM173*, encoding the STING protein, a major adaptor of interferon signaling.[6,63,64] Patients present with cold-aggravated skin lesions that start in the first few weeks of life and skin biopsies confirm vasculitis and vascular occlusion. Lesions heal with tissue loss and scarring and are prominent on acral surfaces, including fingers and toes, the auricular cartilage, tip of the nose and cheeks, and perforation of the nasal septum. Dystrophic nail changes, resorption, and gangrene of fingers and toes are seen. Most patients have hilar or paratracheal and interstitial lung disease with variable severity.[6,65] Patients present with fever and systemic inflammation during flares with increase of the ESR and C-reactive protein level. IgM and C3 depositions can be seen in damaged vessels. Levels of low-titer autoantibodies, such as p-ANCA and c-ANCA, and antiphospholipid antibodies are variable, but do not correlate with the disease activities.[6,65] Later onset and milder phenotypes have been described in 1 report.[63]

Cutaneous manifestations Patients present with early onset skin lesions with a chilblain distribution that are worse on cold exposure. Lesions include telangiectasia; pustular, blistering rashes; vasculitic ulcers; or plaques (**Fig. 4**F) that predominantly developed on cheeks, nose, fingers, toes, and soles of feet. Large eschars and secondary painful crusts on the cheeks and the tip of the helix were reported and are thought to be secondary to localized superinfection of the skin.[6,65]

Dermatopathology On histology, affected skin shows features of small-vessel vasculitis: fibrin deposits and microthrombosis (**Fig. 4**G, H). Skin biopsy samples from some patients show evidence of IgM and C3 depositions.[6] Biopsy of telangiectatic plaques obtained from a patient with SAVI revealed rare epidermal apoptotic keratinocytes and perivascular lymphocytic and neutrophilic infiltrates with nuclear dust (leukocytoclasia) throughout the dermis without damage to the vessel wall, fibrinoid necrosis, and thrombi (**Fig. 4**I). The results of direct immunofluorescence of affected skin were negative.[65]

With severe central nervous system disease

Aicardi-Goutières syndrome Aicardi-Goutières syndrome (AGS) is mostly inherited as a recessive disorder caused by LOF mutations in genes encoding nucleic acid repair enzymes. They include mutations in *TREX1*, a DNA 3′ repair exonuclease 1; *RNASEH2A*, *RNASEH2B*, and *RNASEH2C*, all subunits of ribonuclease H2 enzyme complex; and *SAMHD1*, a cellular enzyme sterile alpha motif (SAM) domain and histidine- aspartic (HD) domain containing protein 1. Autosomal dominant and sporadic forms are caused by heterozygous LOF mutations in *ADAR1*, an RNA repair/editing enzyme, resulting in haploinsufficiency. More variable disease phenotypes are seen with autosomal

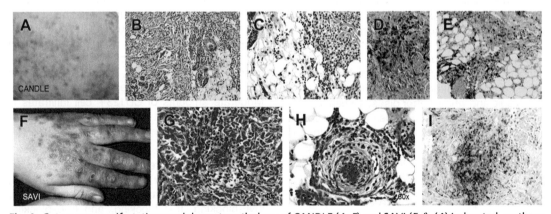

Fig. 4. Cutaneous manifestations and dermatopathology of CANDLE (*A–E*) and SAVI (*F–I*). (*A*) Indurated, erythematous nodule in a patient with CANDLE. (*B*) Deep dermal and subcutaneous inflammatory infiltrates. (*C*) Neutrophil inflammatory infiltrate in subcutaneous adipose tissue. (*D*) MPO+ (neutrophil/myeloid precursor cell in *dark brown*) cell infiltration in interstitium and near blood vessels. (*E*) Perivascular and subcutaneous MPO+ cell infiltrates in CANDLE. (*F*) Violaceous vasculitic plaques on the hand of a patient with SAVI. (*G, H*) Dense inflammatory infiltrate with fibrinoid necrosis of vessel wall and nuclear debris in dermis and subcutis. (*I*) Perivascular and transmural MPO+ cell infiltrate. SAVI, STING- associated vasculopathy with onset in infancy.

dominant GOF mutations in 2 cytosolic dsRNA sensors: *IFIH1* encoding MDA5[5,45] and in *DDX58* encoding RIG-I.[64] AGS is characterized by early onset inflammatory encephalopathy associated with chronic cerebrospinal fluid (CSF) lymphocytosis, and high IFN-alpha levels in the CSF. Brain MRI and computed tomography (CT) findings[66] include intracranial calcifications in the white matter, basal ganglia, and thalami; ischemic or hemorrhagic strokes; white matter loss resulting in cerebral atrophy; and microcephaly. Patients with AGS may present with spasticity; dystonia; large vessel disease, including moyamoya, stenosis, or aneurysms; psychomotor retardation; and death in childhood. Patients may have low titers of autoantibodies. Some patients develop features of autoimmune disorders later in life. Vascular mineral deposits and cortical microinfarctions were occasionally found in postmortem brains. Some heterozygous mutations in *TREX1* and *TMEM173*/STING may cause autosomal dominant forms of sporadic or familial chilblain lupus.

Cutaneous manifestations Cutaneous manifestations include digital vasculitis and or necrosis, chilblains, skin mottling, sometimes with panniculitis, necrotic cheek eruptions, and lipoatrophy.

There is currently no treatment of these patients. Immunotherapy with type I IFN inhibiting agents is being explored.

Deficiency of adenosine deaminase 2 Deficiency of adenosine deaminase 2 (DADA2) is an autosomal recessive disorder caused by compound heterozygous missense mutations in *CECR1*. Patients present with polyarteritis nodosa–like lesions, early onset strokes, peripheral neuropathy, livedo reticularis, and Raynaud symptoms. Other features include hypertension; renal infarct; hepatosplenomegaly; portal hypertension; cervical lymphadenopathy; and systemic manifestations of chronic inflammation, including anemia. There may also be variable low serum immunoglobulin levels with or without autoantibodies.[67–69] Disease severity can vary even within families with the same mutations, ranging from limited skin eruptions to severe fatal systemic vasculitis. MRI may show brain abnormalities, including acute or chronic subcortical lacunar infarct in deep-brain nuclei and the brain stem, indicating small-vessel occlusions.[69] Hemorrhagic strokes, in the context of anticoagulation, have been seen. Some angiographic studies show aneurysms and stenosis of abdominal arteries (mesentery, celiac, hepatic, and renal); renal cortical infarcts or intracranial calcification on brain CT are sometimes seen.[70]

Cutaneous manifestations Cutaneous manifestations include livedo reticularis, skin nodules, purpura (some with leg ulcers), and Raynaud symptoms.

Dermatopathology Histologic findings of skin biopsies include a predominantly interstitial inflammatory infiltrate composed of MPO+ neutrophils and CD68+ macrophages with perivascular CD3+ T lymphocytes,[69] intravascular thrombosis, and necrotizing arterial vasculitis. Nonspecific leukocytoclastic vasculitis and panniculitis in skin biopsies[70] have been reported. In lesional skin and brain biopsies, endothelial damage on staining by anti-CD31 antibodies and endothelial cell activation by E-selectin are seen.

Endothelialization of the hepatic sinusoids in liver biopsy has been reported.[69] In vitro reduced adenosine deaminase 2 (ADA2) activity causes endothelial damage and impaired M2 macrophage differentiation that are hypothesized to lead to vasculopathy and inflammation. An upregulation of interferon-stimulated gene signature in peripheral blood with marked overexpression of neutrophil-derived gene was seen in patients with DADA2.[71]

Treatment Many patients respond to TNF inhibitors but only partially to high doses of glucocorticoids. Fresh frozen plasma and hematopoietic stem cell transplant have been shown to be effective in some patients with deficiency of ADA2. Cytokine inhibitors and cyclophosphamide therapy cannot control severe disease activity. Anticoagulation with aspirin and heparin is not effective; to avoid bleeding complications, anticoagulation is not recommended.

Spondyloenchondrodysplasia with immune dysregulation Spondyloenchondrodysplasia with immune dysregulation (SPENCDI) is caused by recessive LOF mutations in the *ACP5* gene encoding tartrate-resistant phosphatase (TRAP).[72] Lack of TRAP activity leads to hyperphosphorylation and constitutive GOF of osteopontin, a multifunctional protein that plays a role in bone remodeling through osteoclasts and immune regulation through Toll-link receptor 9.[73] Characteristics of this syndrome include short stature; bone dysplasia; and neurologic dysfunction, including spastic paraparesis, seizures, cerebral atrophy, and intracranial calcifications. Many patients developed 3 or more autoimmune diseases during childhood, most commonly systemic lupus erythematosus, thrombocytopenia, antiphospholipid syndrome, hemolytic anemia, hypothyroidism, Sjögren syndrome, and inflammatory myositis. Increased levels of serum IFNα and an upregulation of an IFN signature were noted in patients with SPENCDI. Other features suggesting autoimmune dysregulation include lupus nephritis, arthritis, increased bone mineral density, recurrent respiratory infections, rarely interstitial lung disease, positive antinuclear and anti-dsDNA antibodies, and hypocomplementemia.

Cutaneous manifestations Cutaneous manifestations include palpable purpura, petechiae on the lower limbs, severe eczema, hyperpigmented macules, vitiligo, Raynaud phenomenon with dilated loops of capillaries, livedo reticularis, and sclerodermatous or acrocyanotic changes of hands and feet with edema and digital vasculitis that leads to necrosis and amputation.

Dermatopathology Affected skin biopsies show a perivascular polymorphonuclear infiltrate without evidence of deposition of complement or immunoglobulin, consistent with a nonspecific leukocytoclastic vasculitis.

Treatment Skin lesions are responsive to oral steroid therapy, chloroquine, and cyclophosphamide. Treatment with other immunosuppressive agents, such as azathioprine, mycophenolate mofetil, and rituximab, showed good response.[48,72]

Autoinflammatory Disorders with Granulomatous Skin Lesions

Without significant immunodeficiency

Blau syndrome (pediatric granulomatous arthritis) Blau syndrome (pediatric granulomatous arthritis [PGA]) may be a dominantly inherited GOF mutation in *NOD2/CARD15* and can also present sporadically with a de novo mutation as early onset sarcoidosis. The triad of organ involvement includes skin, eye, and joints. Patients present early in life with fever, ichthyosislike exanthema, and arthritis (**Fig. 5**B) caused by granulomatous synovitis. Ocular manifestations (**Fig. 5**D) include panuveitis, cataract, glaucoma, and permanent vision loss. Other manifestations include sialadenitis, lymphadenopathy, transient neuropathies, granulomatous glomerular and interstitial nephritis, pericarditis, hepatic granulomas, splenic involvement, and chronic renal failure. Laboratory tests show systemic inflammation with leukocytosis, thrombocytosis, and high ESR and CRP level.

Cutaneous manifestations At presentation the rash may appear as generalized erythematous micropapular dermatitis. Later the exanthema becomes tan colored and may present a dirty, scaly appearance. The later stage of the rash lasts longer and develops into a papulonodular (**Fig. 5**A), tender, reddish brown, dirty-looking, and sometimes scaly rash that affects the trunk and the extremities symmetrically. Erythema nodosum–like lesions are also described.

Dermatopathology Histologic findings include an inflammatory infiltrate of typical nonnecrotizing, noncaseating, sarcoid-type granulomas, composed of epithelioid and multinucleated giant cell granulomas that are typically found in the subpapillary dermis or in the vicinity of a hair follicle. The granulomata are referred to as Blau granuloma (**Fig. 5**C). Other findings include leukocytoclastic vasculitis. Noncaseating granulomata are also seen in liver and synovial tissue, but skin biopsies offer a better diagnostic yield.[74]

Treatment Corticosteroids and TNF and IL-1 blockade are used for treatment of severe refractory disease.

With variable features of immunodeficiency and significant central nervous system disease

PLCγ2-associated antibody deficiency and immune dysregulation PLCγ2-associated antibody deficiency and immune dysregulation (PLAID) is an autosomal dominant disorder characterized by urticarial and/or granulomatous skin eruptions, recurrent infections, and positive autoantibodies. A subtype of the disease, autoinflammation and PLCγ2-associated antibody deficiency and immune dysregulation, is dominantly inherited and presents with recurrent erythematous plaques and vesicopustular eruptions, arthralgia, uveitis, and recurrent sinopulmonary infections. Skin biopsies show granuloma.

Other Autoinflammatory Syndromes

LACC1-mediated monogenic Still disease

Laccase domain containing 1 (*LACC1*)-mediated monogenic Still disease is an autosomal recessive form of systemic juvenile idiopathic arthritis associated with homozygous missense mutation of *LACC1*, which encodes laccases, which are multicopper oxidoreductases that catalyze the oxidation of a variety of phenolic and nonphenolic compounds. Patients present with quotidian fever, associated with erythematous maculopapular rash; symmetric polyarthritis affecting small and large joints; and sometimes with tenosynovitis, serositis, organomegaly, and lymphadenopathy. Laboratory findings include leukocytosis, thrombocytosis, and increased levels of acute phase reactants. Some patients have positive ANA, weak rheumatoid factor, but no extractable nuclear antigen. Erosive arthritic changes with joint destruction can be seen on imaging studies. The disease is refractory to different immunosuppressive agents: NSAIDs; systemic corticosteroids;

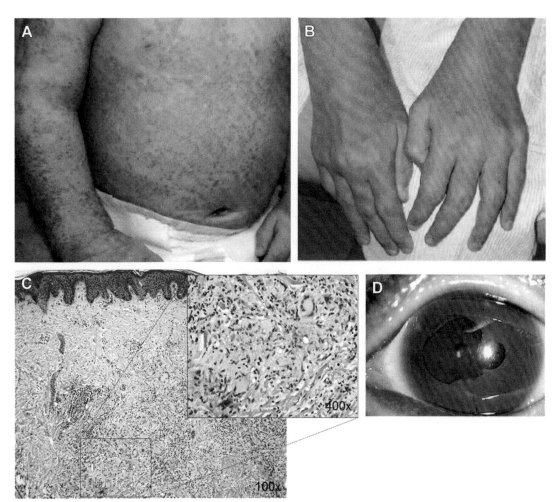

Fig. 5. PGA or Blau syndrome. (*A*) Numerous 1-mm to 2-mm, red-brown to pinkish tan, flat-topped papules on the trunk and extremities. (*B*) Nonerosive arthritis. (*C*) Histology of skin biopsy shows chronic granulomatous inflammation in dermis, with multiple nonnecrotizing granulomas and scattered lymphocytes throughout the dermis. The overlying epidemics is unremarkable and the papillary dermis is uninvolved. The nonnecrotizing (sarcoid type) granulomas are composed of histiocytes/tissue macrophages with multinucleated giant cells and a peripheral rim of lymphocytes (original magnification, ×100 [inset: original magnification, ×400]). (*D*) Anterior synechiae in a patient with Blau syndrome who had a cataract with chronic uveitis.

methotrexate; and biologic agents, including etanercept, adalimumab, tocilizumab, and rituximab.[75]

SUMMARY

Monogenic autoinflammatory disorders are caused by dysregulation in innate immune pathways that coordinate immune responses to intracellular and extracellular danger signals. Many autoinflammatory diseases mimic infections or sepsis, particularly early in life, and rapidly progress to organ damage and death, which makes it imperative to diagnose these conditions early to ensure early appropriate treatment. Most monogenic autoinflammatory disorders present with

neutrophilic dermatoses and a careful clinical and histopathologic evaluation of the skin findings often presents the first clue to a specific diagnosis. The presence of mutations in genes that encode proteins that enuclate inflammasomes and regulate IL-1β has led to the use and approval of IL-1 blocking agents in CAPS. Recently mutations in genes that regulate nucleic acid metabolism and viral sensing leading to increased type-I IFN production have suggested a role of IFN blocking agents in treating these conditions. Other cytokine amplification loops include IL-17 in the skin and IL-18 in the context of the risk of developing MAS. With therapies targeting dysregulated innate immune pathways becoming increasingly available, a personalized treatment approach becomes possible. Furthermore, the discovery of novel monogenic genetic diseases points to inflammatory pathways that are dysregulated in more common, genetically complex inflammatory diseases and may lead to the discovery of key regulators in innate immune pathways that can become targets for therapeutic intervention.

REFERENCES

1. de Jesus AA, Canna SW, Liu Y, et al. Molecular mechanisms in genetically defined autoinflammatory diseases: disorders of amplified danger signaling. Annu Rev Immunol 2015;33:823–74.
2. French FMF Consortium. A candidate gene for familial Mediterranean fever. Nat Genet 1997;17(1): 25–31.
3. Localization of the familial Mediterranean fever gene (FMF) to a 250-kb interval in non-Ashkenazi Jewish founder haplotypes. The French FMF Consortium. Am J Hum Genet 1996;59(3):603–12.
4. McDermott MF, Aksentijevich I, Galon J, et al. Germline mutations in the extracellular domains of the 55 kDa TNF receptor, TNFR1, define a family of dominantly inherited autoinflammatory syndromes. Cell 1999;97(1):133–44.
5. Rutsch F, MacDougall M, Lu C, et al. A specific IFIH1 gain-of-function mutation causes Singleton-Merten syndrome. Am J Hum Genet 2015;96(2): 275–82.
6. Liu Y, Jesus AA, Marrero B, et al. Activated STING in a vascular and pulmonary syndrome. N Engl J Med 2014;371(6):507–18.
7. Onen F. Familial Mediterranean fever. Rheumatol Int 2006;26(6):489–96.
8. Takahashi T, Fujisawa T, Kimura M, et al. Familial Mediterranean fever variant with repeated atypical skin eruptions. J Dermatol 2015;42(9):903–5.
9. Majeed HA, Quabazard Z, Hijazi Z, et al. The cutaneous manifestations in children with familial Mediterranean fever (recurrent hereditary polyserositis). A six-year study. Q J Med 1990;75(278):607–16.
10. Barzilai A, Langevitz P, Goldberg I, et al. Erysipelas-like erythema of familial Mediterranean fever: clinico-pathologic correlation. J Am Acad Dermatol 2000; 42(5 Pt 1):791–5.
11. Azizi E, Fisher BK. Cutaneous manifestations of familial Mediterranean fever. Arch Dermatol 1976; 112(3):364–6.
12. Cuisset L, Drenth JP, Simon A, et al. Molecular analysis of MVK mutations and enzymatic activity in hyper-IgD and periodic fever syndrome. Eur J Hum Genet 2001;9(4):260–6.
13. Braun-Falco M, Ruzicka T. Skin manifestations in autoinflammatory syndromes. J Dtsch Dermatol Ges 2011;9(3):232–46.
14. van der Hilst JC, Bodar EJ, Barron KS, et al. Long-term follow-up, clinical features, and quality of life in a series of 103 patients with hyperimmunoglobulinemia D syndrome. Medicine 2008;87(6):301–10.
15. Boom BW, Daha MR, Vermeer BJ, et al. IgD immune complex vasculitis in a patient with hyperimmunoglobulinemia D and periodic fever. Arch Dermatol 1990;126(12):1621–4.
16. ter Haar NM, Oswald M, Jeyaratnam J, et al. Recommendations for the management of autoinflammatory diseases. Ann Rheum Dis 2015;74(9):1636–44.
17. Siegel RM, Muppidi J, Roberts M, et al. Death receptor signaling and autoimmunity. Immunol Res 2003;27(2–3):499–512.
18. Bulua AC, Simon A, Maddipati R, et al. Mitochondrial reactive oxygen species promote production of proinflammatory cytokines and are elevated in TNFR1-associated periodic syndrome (TRAPS). J Exp Med 2011;208(3):519–33.
19. Nakamura M, Kobayashi M, Tokura Y. A novel missense mutation in tumour necrosis factor receptor superfamily 1A (TNFRSF1A) gene found in tumour necrosis factor receptor-associated periodic syndrome (TRAPS) manifesting adult-onset Still disease-like skin eruptions: report of a case and review of the Japanese patients. Br J Dermatol 2009; 161(4):968–70.
20. Hull KM, Wong K, Wood GM, et al. Monocytic fasciitis: a newly recognized clinical feature of tumor necrosis factor receptor dysfunction. Arthritis Rheum 2002;46(8):2189–94.
21. Gattorno M, Pelagatti MA, Meini A, et al. Persistent efficacy of anakinra in patients with tumor necrosis factor receptor-associated periodic syndrome. Arthritis Rheum 2008;58(5):1516–20.
22. Sacre K, Brihaye B, Lidove O, et al. Dramatic improvement following interleukin 1beta blockade in tumor necrosis factor receptor-1-associated syndrome (TRAPS) resistant to anti-TNF-alpha therapy. J Rheumatol 2008;35(2):357–8.
23. Hoffman HM, Mueller JL, Broide DH, et al. Mutation of a new gene encoding a putative pyrin-like protein causes familial cold autoinflammatory syndrome and Muckle-Wells syndrome. Nat Genet 2001; 29(3):301–5.
24. Agostini L, Martinon F, Burns K, et al. NALP3 forms an IL-1beta-processing inflammasome with increased activity in Muckle-Wells autoinflammatory disorder. Immunity 2004;20(3):319–25.
25. Canna SW, de Jesus AA, Gouni S, et al. An activating NLRC4 inflammasome mutation causes autoinflammation with recurrent macrophage activation syndrome. Nat Genet 2014;46(10):1140–6.
26. Romberg N, Al Moussawi K, Nelson-Williams C, et al. Mutation of NLRC4 causes a syndrome of enterocolitis and autoinflammation. Nat Genet 2014;46(10):1135–9.

27. Shimizu M, Nakagishi Y, Inoue N, et al. Interleukin-18 for predicting the development of macrophage activation syndrome in systemic juvenile idiopathic arthritis. Clin Immunol 2015;160(2):277–81.

28. Ichida H, Kawaguchi Y, Sugiura T, et al. Clinical manifestations of Adult-onset Still's disease presenting with erosive arthritis: association with low levels of ferritin and interleukin-18. Arthritis Care Res 2014;66(4):642–6.

29. Kitamura A, Sasaki Y, Abe T, et al. An inherited mutation in NLRC4 causes autoinflammation in human and mice. J Exp Med 2014;211(12):2385–96.

30. Aksentijevich I, Masters SL, Ferguson PJ, et al. An autoinflammatory disease with deficiency of the interleukin-1-receptor antagonist. N Engl J Med 2009;360(23):2426–37.

31. Minkis K, Aksentijevich I, Goldbach-Mansky R, et al. Interleukin 1 receptor antagonist deficiency presenting as infantile pustulosis mimicking infantile pustular psoriasis. Arch Dermatol 2012;148(6):747–52.

32. Reddy S, Jia S, Geoffrey R, et al. An autoinflammatory disease due to homozygous deletion of the IL1RN locus. N Engl J Med 2009;360(23):2438–44.

33. Ferguson PJ, Chen S, Tayeh MK, et al. Homozygous mutations in LPIN2 are responsible for the syndrome of chronic recurrent multifocal osteomyelitis and congenital dyserythropoietic anaemia (Majeed syndrome). J Med Genet 2005;42(7):551–7.

34. Majeed HA, Kalaawi M, Mohanty D, et al. Congenital dyserythropoietic anemia and chronic recurrent multifocal osteomyelitis in three related children and the association with Sweet syndrome in two siblings. J Pediatr 1989;115(5 Pt 1):730–4.

35. Herlin T, Fiirgaard B, Bjerre M, et al. Efficacy of anti-IL-1 treatment in Majeed syndrome. Ann Rheum Dis 2013;72(3):410–3.

36. Schnellbacher C, Ciocca G, Menendez R, et al. Deficiency of interleukin-1 receptor antagonist responsive to anakinra. Pediatr Dermatol 2013;30(6):758–60.

37. El-Shanti H, Ferguson P. Majeed syndrome. In: Pagon RA, Adam MP, Ardinger HH, et al, editors. Seattle (WA): GeneReviews; 1993.

38. Wise CA, Gillum JD, Seidman CE, et al. Mutations in CD2BP1 disrupt binding to PTP PEST and are responsible for PAPA syndrome, an autoinflammatory disorder. Hum Mol Genet 2002;11(8):961–9.

39. Zhou Q, Wang H, Schwartz DM, et al. Loss-of-function mutations in TNFAIP3 leading to A20 haploinsufficiency cause an early-onset autoinflammatory disease. Nat Genet 2016;48(1):67–73.

40. Li H, Liu Q, Hou S, et al. TNFAIP3 gene polymorphisms confer risk for Behcet's disease in a Chinese Han population. Hum Genet 2013;132(3):293–300.

41. Demirkesen C, Tuzuner N, Mat C, et al. Clinicopathologic evaluation of nodular cutaneous lesions of Behcet syndrome. Am J Clin Pathol 2001;116(3):341–6.

42. Tortola L, Rosenwald E, Abel B, et al. Psoriasiform dermatitis is driven by IL-36-mediated DC-keratinocyte crosstalk. J Clin Invest 2012;122(11):3965–76.

43. Marrakchi S, Guigue P, Renshaw BR, et al. Interleukin-36-receptor antagonist deficiency and generalized pustular psoriasis. N Engl J Med 2011;365(7):620–8.

44. Harden JL, Lewis SM, Pierson KC, et al. CARD14 expression in dermal endothelial cells in psoriasis. PLoS One 2014;9(11):e111255.

45. Bursztejn AC, Briggs TA, del Toro Duany Y, et al. Unusual cutaneous features associated with a heterozygous gain-of-function mutation in IFIH1: overlap between Aicardi-Goutieres and Singleton-Merten syndromes. Br J Dermatol 2015;173(6):1505–13.

46. Isailovic N, Daigo K, Mantovani A, et al. Interleukin-17 and innate immunity in infections and chronic inflammation. J Autoimmun 2015;60:1–11.

47. Reynolds JM, Angkasekwinai P, Dong C. IL-17 family member cytokines: regulation and function in innate immunity. Cytokine Growth Factor Rev 2010;21(6):413–23.

48. Lausch E, Janecke A, Bros M, et al. Genetic deficiency of tartrate-resistant acid phosphatase associated with skeletal dysplasia, cerebral calcifications and autoimmunity. Nat Genet 2011;43(2):132–7.

49. Campa M, Mansouri B, Warren R, et al. A review of biologic therapies targeting IL-23 and IL-17 for use in moderate-to-severe plaque psoriasis. Dermatol Ther 2016;6(1):1–12.

50. Glocker EO, Kotlarz D, Boztug K, et al. Inflammatory bowel disease and mutations affecting the interleukin-10 receptor. N Engl J Med 2009;361(21):2033–45.

51. Shouval DS, Biswas A, Goettel JA, et al. Interleukin-10 receptor signaling in innate immune cells regulates mucosal immune tolerance and anti-inflammatory macrophage function. Immunity 2014;40(5):706–19.

52. Moore KW, de Waal Malefyt R, Coffman RL, et al. Interleukin-10 and the interleukin-10 receptor. Annu Rev Immunol 2001;19:683–765.

53. Briggs TA, Rice GI, Adib N, et al. Spondyloenchondrodysplasia due to mutations in ACP5: a comprehensive survey. J Clin Immunol 2016;36(3):220–34.

54. Brehm A, Liu Y, Sheikh A, et al. Additive loss-of-function proteasome subunit mutations in CANDLE/PRAAS patients promote type I IFN production. J Clin Invest 2016;126(2):795.

55. Tufekci O, Bengoa S, Karapinar TH, et al. CANDLE syndrome: a recently described autoinflammatory syndrome. J Pediatr Hematol Oncol 2015;37(4):296–9.

56. Agarwal AK, Xing C, DeMartino GN, et al. PSMB8 encoding the beta5i proteasome subunit is mutated in joint contractures, muscle atrophy, microcytic anemia, and panniculitis-induced lipodystrophy syndrome. Am J Hum Genet 2010;87(6):866–72.

57. Kanazawa N, Arima K, Ida H, et al. Nakajo-Nishimura syndrome. Nihon Rinsho Meneki Gakkai Kaishi 2011;34(5):388–400.

58. Arima K, Kinoshita A, Mishima H, et al. Proteasome assembly defect due to a proteasome subunit beta type 8 (PSMB8) mutation causes the autoinflammatory disorder, Nakajo-Nishimura syndrome. Proc Natl Acad Sci U S A 2011;108(36):14914–9.

59. Kitamura A, Maekawa Y, Uehara H, et al. A mutation in the immunoproteasome subunit PSMB8 causes autoinflammation and lipodystrophy in humans. J Clin Invest 2011;121(10):4150–60.

60. Liu Y, Ramot Y, Torrelo A, et al. Mutations in proteasome subunit beta type 8 cause chronic atypical neutrophilic dermatosis with lipodystrophy and elevated temperature with evidence of genetic and phenotypic heterogeneity. Arthritis Rheum 2012; 64(3):895–907.

61. Torrelo A, Colmenero I, Requena L, et al. Histologic and immunohistochemical features of the skin lesions in CANDLE syndrome. Am J Dermatopathol 2015;37(7):517–22.

62. Almeida de Jesus A, Goldbach-Mansky R. Monogenic autoinflammatory diseases: concept and clinical manifestations. Clin Immunol 2013;147(3):155–74.

63. Jeremiah N, Neven B, Gentili M, et al. Inherited STING-activating mutation underlies a familial inflammatory syndrome with lupus-like manifestations. J Clin Invest 2014;124(12):5516–20.

64. Crow YJ, Manel N. Aicardi-Goutieres syndrome and the type I interferonopathies. Nat Rev Immunol 2015; 15(7):429–40.

65. Munoz J, Rodiere M, Jeremiah N, et al. Stimulator of interferon genes-associated vasculopathy with onset in infancy: a mimic of childhood granulomatosis with polyangiitis. JAMA Dermatol 2015;151(8): 872–7.

66. La Piana R, Uggetti C, Roncarolo F, et al. Neuroradiologic patterns and novel imaging findings in Aicardi-Goutieres syndrome. Neurology 2016;86(1): 28–35.

67. Kastner DL, Zhou Q, Aksentijevich I. Mutant ADA2 in vasculopathies. N Engl J Med 2014;371(5):480–1.

68. Segel R, King MC, Levy-Lahad E. Mutant ADA2 in vasculopathies. N Engl J Med 2014;371(5):481.

69. Zhou Q, Yang D, Ombrello AK, et al. Early-onset stroke and vasculopathy associated with mutations in ADA2. N Engl J Med 2014;370(10):911–20.

70. Navon Elkan P, Pierce SB, Segel R, et al. Mutant adenosine deaminase 2 in a polyarteritis nodosa vasculopathy. N Engl J Med 2014;370(10):921–31.

71. Belot A, Wassmer E, Twilt M, et al. Mutations in CECR1 associated with a neutrophil signature in peripheral blood. Pediatr Rheumatol Online J 2014;12:44.

72. Briggs TA, Rice GI, Daly S, et al. Tartrate-resistant acid phosphatase deficiency causes a bone dysplasia with autoimmunity and a type I interferon expression signature. Nat Genet 2011;43(2):127–31.

73. Shinohara ML, Lu L, Bu J, et al. Osteopontin expression is essential for interferon-alpha production by plasmacytoid dendritic cells. Nat Immunol 2006; 7(5):498–506.

74. Wouters CH, Maes A, Foley KP, et al. Blau syndrome, the prototypic auto-inflammatory granulomatous disease. Pediatr Rheumatol Online J 2014;12:33.

75. Wakil SM, Monies DM, Abouelhoda M, et al. Association of a mutation in LACC1 with a monogenic form of systemic juvenile idiopathic arthritis. Arthritis Rheumatol 2015;67(1):288–95.

The Critical and Multifunctional Roles of Antimicrobial Peptides in Dermatology

Toshiya Takahashi, MD, PhD, Richard L. Gallo, MD, PhD*

KEYWORDS

- Antimicrobial peptides • Cathelicidin • Defensins • Immunology • Rosacea • Psoriasis
- Atopic dermatitis

KEY POINTS

- Antimicrobial peptides (AMPs) not only kill bacteria but also control inflammation and other host responses.
- The main AMPs that are secreted in skin are cathelicidin and human β-defensins.
- Cathelicidin and β-defensins are 2 of many families of antimicrobial peptides in the skin that increase in response to injury.
- In psoriatic and rosacea skin, AMPs are overexpressed and promote inflammation. On the other hand, in atopic dermatitis, some AMPs fail to be appropriately induced and enable infection.
- Control of the expression and action of AMPs can be of therapeutic benefit for skin diseases.

INTRODUCTION

Skin is the physical and immunologic armor of the body. Both the physical and immune defense system of the skin combine to accomplish functions essential to life, including preventing invasion by pathogenic microbes such as bacteria, fungi, viruses, and parasites, and maintaining homeostasis with commensal microorganisms. Antimicrobial peptides and proteins (AMPs) have an essential role in this immunologic armor and enable epithelial surfaces to cope with many microbial challenges. They are evolutionarily ancient innate immune effectors that are produced by almost all plants and animals.[1] More than 1800 AMPs have been identified and more than 20 AMPs have been found in skin.[2] They typically are small (12–50 amino acids residues), have positive charge and amphipathic structure,[2] features that allow them to interact with negatively charged phospholipid head groups and hydrophobic fatty acid chains of microbial membranes, and kill some organisms by disrupting the microbial membrane and release of cytosol components.[3,4]

However, AMPs are not only natural antibiotics. Recently, common human skin disorders such as rosacea, psoriasis, and atopic dermatitis (AD) have been linked to an abnormality of AMPs. These skin diseases cannot be attributed only to microorganisms. Contrary to the term antimicrobial, AMPs not only directly kill or inhibit the growth of microorganisms[5] but also modify host inflammatory responses by a variety of mechanisms, including action as chemotactic agents, angiogenic factors,

Funding Sources: R.L. Gallo receives funding from the NIH through grants R01AI116576, R01AR064781, R01AI052453, R21AR0675478, U19AI117673 and P01HL107150.
Conflict of Interest: None.
Department of Dermatology, University of California, San Diego, La Jolla, CA 92093, USA
* Corresponding author.
E-mail address: rgallo@ucsd.edu

Dermatol Clin 35 (2017) 39–50
http://dx.doi.org/10.1016/j.det.2016.07.006
0733-8635/17/© 2016 Elsevier Inc. All rights reserved.

derm.theclinics.com

Abbreviations and acronyms

AD	Atopic dermatitis
AMP	Antimicrobial peptide
DAMPs	Danger or Damage-associated molecular patterns
FPRL1	Formyl peptide receptor-like 1
hBD	Human β-defensin
HIV	Human immunodeficiency virus
IFN	Interferon
IL	Interleukin
KLK	Kallikrein
MCET	Mast cell extracellular trap
mDC	Myeloid dendritic cells
pDC	Plasmacytoid dendritic cell
PSMγ	Phenol-soluble modulin-γ
Th cells	T-helper cells
TLR	Toll-like receptor
TNF	Tumor necrosis factor
UV	Ultraviolet
VDRE	Vitamin D response element

and regulators of cell proliferation.[2] This article summarizes how they participate in human skin diseases and what the knowledge of AMPs will do for clinical dermatology.

ANTIMICROBIAL PROTEIN FUNCTION: BASIC

Key AMPs of the skin's repertoire are the catheclicidins, the first AMP discovered in mammalian skin[6] and β-defensins.[7] The single cathelicidin gene (CAMP) encodes a precursor protein, hCAP18 in humans.[8] This protein can be alternatively cleaved to generate several active AMPs, including the 37-amino-acid peptide LL-37.[9] In contrast to cathelicidin, approximately 90 β-defensin genes have been identified in mice and humans. Both cathelicidins and β-defensins are antimicrobial against a diverse range of skin pathogens, including gram-negative and gram-positive bacteria, fungi, viruses, and parasites.[2] In normal skin, keratinocytes produce various AMPs at lower levels to defend the skin barrier,[10] whereas cathelicidin precursor protein and mature peptide are the most abundantly expressed by resident mast cells.[11] Mast cells normally occupy positions around blood vessels and store large amounts of cathelicidin in preformed granules. This localization places the AMPs derived from mast cells in an ideal position to resist infections after skin injury and inoculation with pathogens.[12] Moreover, AMPs has been detected in mast cell extracellular traps (MCETs).[13] Once inflamed, skin produces cathelicidin through increased expression of CAP18 by keratinocytes, adipocytes,[14]

and increased local deposition by recruited neutrophils.[15–17]

Though many AMPs target essential cell wall or cell membrane structures through enzymatic or nonenzymatic disruption, AMPs can also function as potent immune regulators by signaling through chemokine receptors and by inhibiting or enhancing Toll-like receptor (TLR) signaling.[18] AMPs seem to function not only under stimulus from pathogen-associated molecular patterns but also as triggered by danger-associated or damage-associated molecular patterns, including urea[19] and nucleic acids.[20] This means that AMPs are not only antimicrobial.

The expression, secretion, and activity of most AMPs are tightly controlled. Cathelicidins are synthesized as propeptides. Serine proteases are responsible for the processing of cathelicidins into various sizes. In neutrophils, the propeptide is removed by proteinase 3,[21] whereas processing is carried out by kallikreins (KLKs, also known as stratum corneum tryptic enzyme) in keratinocytes.[22] Interestingly, the antimicrobial activity of cathelicidin peptides differs by their size.[23] Processing mechanisms generate the active forms of AMPs in skin and the mechanism is useful to prevent potential harmful effects of these proteins on mammalian cell membranes.[24] A particularly surprising observation came with the recognition that the human cathelicidin gene is under transcriptional control of a vitamin D response element (VDRE).[25,26] Following skin injury or infection, $25(OH)D3$ is hydroxylated by the enzyme cytochrome p450, 27B1 (CYP27B1) to $1,25(OH)_2D3$, and this is stimulated locally by activation of TLR2 or local cytokines such as tumor necrosis factor (TNF) or type I interferons (IFNs).[27,28] This local enzymatic event enables rapid induction of CAMP expression through binding of $1,25(OH)_2D3$ to the VDRE. These observations suggest that AMP expression could be influenced by serum vitamin D level,[29] dietary vitamin D,[30] or vitamin D generated by exposure of the skin to sunlight.[31] This implies that the nutritional environment is probably a source of important signals that control AMP expression. Conversely, LL-37 also transactivates epidermal growth factor receptor and downstream signaling in epithelial cells.[32,33]

Similarly, β-defensins are expressed as propeptides; however, the processing mechanism remains to be established.[34]

ANTIMICROBIAL PROTEIN FUNCTION IN VIVO

AMPs not only provide resistance to infection by killing bacteria but may also determine microbiota composition and limit access of the microbiota to host tissues. Surprisingly, an important component of the surface antimicrobial shield of the skin is produced by the resident microorganisms themselves. Gram-positive bacteria such as *Lactococcus*, *Streptococcus*, and *Streptomyces* spp produce factors, known as bacteriocins, that are another type of AMP and inhibit the growth of other bacterial strains and species that could compete for nutrients and other resources. *Staphylococcus epidermidis*, the dominant bacterium cultured from the skin microflora, produces another type of AMP, phenol-soluble modulin (PSM)-γ. PSMγ causes membrane leakage in target bacteria, which indicates that they function in a manner similar to that of host-derived AMPs.[35] Interestingly, PSMs are functional in vivo; nanomolar concentrations decreased the survival of group A streptococcus on normal human skin but did not affect the survival of *S epidermidis* from which the peptide was derived. In addition, PSMs enhance the capacity of bacterial killing activity by human neutrophils by inducing their neutrophil extracellular traps.[35] This implies human innate immune systems cooperate with commensal bacteria to balance the microbiome via those AMPs. Another important example of the protective action of *S epidermidis* in vivo was observed on the surface of the nasal cavity. Nasal colonization by *S aureus* was inhibited in individuals who were colonized with specific strains of *S epidermidis* that produced a serine protease with the capacity to destroy biofilms formed by *S aureus*.[36] Hence, a thiolactone-containing peptide produced by *S epidermidis* blocks the *S aureus* quorum-sensing system that controls the production of various virulence factors.[37] Thus, the selective activity of AMPs produced by commensal organisms may be an important part of a normal host defense strategy against pathogen colonization and microbe-derived AMPs probably work together with host-derived proteins to establish the composition of the skin surface microbiome.

ANTIMICROBIAL PROTEINS AND HUMAN SKIN DISEASE
Rosacea

The pathogenesis of rosacea is complex. Emotional stress, spicy foods, hot beverages, alcohol consumption, high environmental temperatures, sun exposure, and menopause exacerbate rosacea symptoms such as erythema, rash, and telangiectasia.[38] These findings implied that the external environment would affect rosacea but they are not sufficient or specific to rosacea. In other words, specific intrinsic factors in the host that recognizes and responds to the diverse environmental triggers must be the key to understanding the pathogenesis of rosacea. In innate immunity, the pattern recognition system responds to those environmental stimuli. Triggering the innate immune system normally leads to a controlled increase in cytokines and antimicrobial molecules in the skin, including cathelicidin.[16,39,40] Some forms of cathelicidin peptides have a unique capacity to be both vasoactive and proinflammatory.[23,41] A key to understanding rosacea came with the observation that individuals with rosacea expressed abnormally high levels of cathelicidin in their epidermis.[42] Importantly, the cathelicidin peptide forms found in rosacea were not only more abundant but were also different in molecular weights compared with those in normal individuals. These abnormal cathelicidin peptides promote and regulate leukocyte chemotaxis,[43] angiogenesis,[41] and expression of extracellular matrix components,[6] whereas the types commonly found on normal skin function mostly as antibiotics and have little to no action in inflammation.[23,44] Normally, active form LL-37 is typically present in neutrophils recruited to infected or injured skin; however, in the case of rosacea patients, LL-37 seems to be generated in the epidermis by an abnormal action of serine proteases. When LL-37 was applied in animal models, it was found to be a potent angiogenic factor and resulted in neovascularization in a rabbit model of hind-limb ischemia.[41] Angiogenesis by LL-37 is mediated by formyl peptide receptor-like 1, a G-protein-coupled receptor expressed on endothelial cells.[41] Moreover, epidermal growth factor receptor signaling, which is in part induced by AMPs, induces vascular endothelial growth factor in epidermal keratinocytes.[45] Yamasaki and colleagues[42] reported that injection of cathelicidin or the enzymes that produce cathelicidin into mice skin resulted in skin inflammation resembling pathologic changes in rosacea. Abnormal production of local serine protease KLK5, which processes cathelicidin peptides from a precursor protein in the epidermis, is a cause for the presence of abundant cathelicidin peptides.[22] This suggests that the abnormally high protease activity found in rosacea patients results in abnormal processing cathelicidin to peptides that induce the characteristic inflammation and vascular changes of rosacea (**Fig. 1**).

Why do individuals prone to rosacea react with high KLK5 and cathelicidin? A potential explanation for this response can be found by understanding that the innate immune system of the skin is programmed to detect microbes, tissue damage such as ultraviolet (UV)-induced apoptosis, or damage of the extracellular matrix.[46,47] TLRs are

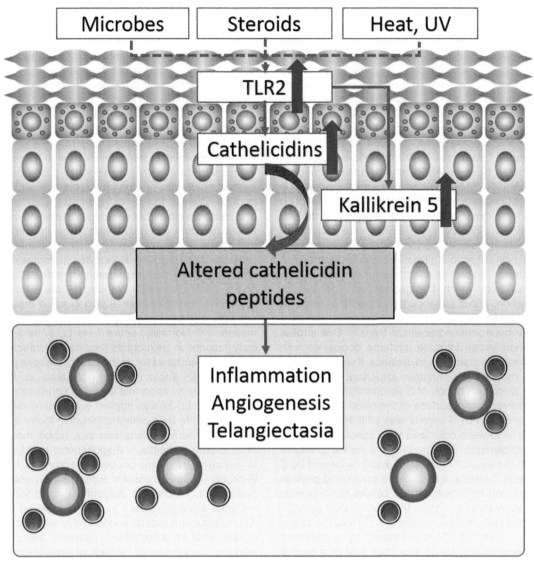

Fig. 1. Rosacea skin is susceptible to environmental changes, altered hormone balance, and microbe challenges because of increased Toll-like receptor 2 (TLR2). The activation of TLR2 then induces an increase in effector molecules: cathelicidin and kallikrein 5 (KLK5). Elevated KLK5 results in generation of active peptides such as LL-37. This peptide stimulates vascular changes and inflammatory cell recruitment.

a major and potent mechanism that broadly recognizes microbe derivatives and induces cellular responses such as cytokines and AMPs. In the skin of individuals with rosacea, TLR2 is more highly expressed compared with nonaffected individuals.[48] Increased TLR2 enhances skin susceptibility to specific environmental stimuli and leads to increased cathelicidin production. Cathelicidin transcription in epidermal keratinocytes is also regulated by the active form of vitamin D 1,25(OH)$_2$D3.[49] TLR2 stimulation amplifies 1,25(OH)$_2$D3 by increasing enzymatic conversion from the inactive form found in the diet

and generated by UV exposure.[27,28] In turn, increased 1,25(OH)$_2$D3 enables the epidermis to produce more cathelicidin antimicrobial peptides. KLK5 mRNA transcription is also increased by 1,25(OH)$_2$D3 keratinocytes.[50] Actually, increasing or stimulating TLR2 increased KLK5, whereas knocking out TLR2 decreased KLK5.[48] These findings, therefore, suggest that the increase of TLR2 in rosacea skin makes the skin of these patients susceptible to microbes and environmental stimuli, resulting in high cathelicidin and KLK5 expression that then evokes the disease. Interestingly, it is reported that glucocorticoids increase TLR2 expression in epidermal keratinocytes.[51] This may imply that glucocorticoid-induced rosacea-like dermatitis, so-called perioral dermatitis, includes erythema, pustules, and papules somewhat similar to those seen in rosacea, may be caused via TLR2. Finally, many of the current therapies for rosacea can be explained via this pathway. Topical and oral retinoids not only induce connective tissue remodeling but also downregulate TLR2.[52,53] Azelaic acid decreases the expression of KLK5 and cathelicidin.[54] And doxycycline has anti-inflammatory function via decrease of KLK5 activity by inhibiting matrix metalloproteinases.[55] Recently, Muto and colleagues[56] reported that mast cells (MCs)-deficient (KitW-sh) mice did not develop rosacea-like features after LL-37 injection into the dermis and that stabilization of mast cells can directly reduce skin inflammation in mice and rosacea patients. These results highlight the important role of mast cells in the development of inflammation after cathelicidin activation and the possibility of downregulation of activated mast cells for a therapy for rosacea. In vivo, Two and colleagues[57] described that inhibition of KLK5 may improve the clinical signs of rosacea by decreasing LL-37 production. A turning point of rosacea therapy may have been reached.

Psoriasis

Psoriasis is neither an exclusive epidermal disease nor a pure T-cell–mediated disorder. Clearly, T cell responses are critical, including the contribution of both T-helper (Th)1 and Th17 cells to promote inflammation by producing cytokines, including TNF-α, IFN-γ, interleukin (IL)-12, IL-17A, IL-22, and IL-23.[58] However, epidermal keratinocytes within the epidermis of psoriatic plaques are also abnormal in many aspects and likely influence immunocytes by production of inflammatory cytokines and chemokines.[59] One of the abnormalities of keratinocytes in psoriasis is the excessive production of AMPs.[60,61] Harder and colleagues[7,62] isolated human β-defensin (hBD)2 and hBD3, which are only induced by stimulation with proinflammatory cytokines and microbial products,[2] and from psoriatic scales. β-defensin gene copy numbers have been associated with the severity of psoriasis.[63] TNF-α and IFN-γ, which are highly expressed in psoriatic lesions, induce hBD2 and hBD3 expression in keratinocytes.[7,64] In addition, Th17 cytokines, IL-17A and IL-22 are also inducers of hBD2.[65] The role for hBD in the pathogenesis of psoriasis is not fully understood. However, recently Lande and colleagues[66] reported that hBD2, hBD3, and lysozyme can activate plasmacytoid dendritic cells (pDCs) by themselves and in cooperation with LL-37.

Among the 21 S-100 proteins, S100A7 (psoriasin), S100A8 (calgranulin A), S100A9 (calgranulin B), S100A12 (calgranulin C), and S100A15 have some antimicrobial activity.[60] These are all abundantly expressed in psoriatic lesions or are elevated in serum from psoriatic patients. S100A7, psoriasin, has been best studied because this protein was first discovered in psoriatic skin lesions.[67] This molecule is induced by calcium, vitamin D, retinoic acid, microbial products, TNF-α, IL-17A, and IL-22,[3,65,68–70] and is thought to have a chemotactic role in psoriasis.[71]

Cathelicidin has been highlighted as a modulator of psoriasis development. The upregulation of LL-37 expression in psoriatic epidermis was reported first in 1997.[15] Afterward, it has been shown that the abundance of AMPs including LL-37 and hBD2 in psoriatic lesions is associated with a low rate of infection.[72] In 2007, Lande and colleagues[73] demonstrated an important immune-modulatory function for LL-37 in psoriasis. LL-37 can drive inflammation in psoriasis through its capacity to enable pDCs to recognize self-DNA through TLR9. This response is different from the classical concept that TLR9 recognizes unmethylated DNA sequences (CpG dinucleotides) found in microbial DNA[74] and, in turn, serves as an innate immunity warning system against infection. This activation induces a large amount of type I IFN production, leading to myeloid dendritic cells (mDCs) activation, Th1/Th17 differentiation, and keratinocyte activation.[58] The involvement of type I IFN in the pathogenesis of psoriasis has been suggested by several studies[75–77] and type I IFNs have been reported to activate autoimmune T cells through the maturation of DCs.[78] pDCs are thought to be major type I IFN-producing cells, and produce many IFN-α in psoriasis[79]; however, Morizane and colleagues[80] has demonstrated that LL-37 and DNA activation of keratinocytes also greatly increases type I IFN production through TLR9. Therefore, the main source of type I IFNs must be reconsidered again because there are more keratinocytes than pDCs in skin, and because keratinocytes are in more superficial site with greater direct contact to genomic DNA and other external stimuli known to exacerbate inflammation. This may be relevant to the Köbner phenomenon seen in psoriasis, in which clinical exacerbation is caused by minor superficial injury of the epidermis. LL-37 secretion and following IFN production via TLR9 activation may explain this phenomenon. Furthermore, LL-37 has also forms complexes with self-RNA, leading to the activation of TLR7 in pDCs and TLR8 in mDCs in psoriasis[81] (Fig. 2). Moreover, in search of a DC type that specifically accumulates in psoriatic skin lesion and has proinflammatory function, Lowes and

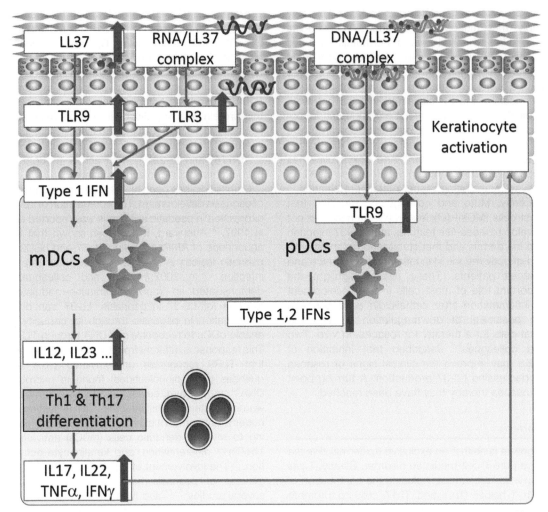

Fig. 2. Psoriasis and cathelicidins. Stressed cells stimulated by trauma or bacterial products release LL-37, self-RNA and self-DNA. Self-RNA and self-DNA form complexes with LL-37 and the complexes are then recognized by Toll-like TLR9 in plasmacytoid dendritic cells (pDCs). On the other hand, LL-37 induces TLR9 expression in keratinocytes (KCs) and greatly enhances type I IFN production induced by TLR3 and 9 signaling. Stimulated mDCs induce the differentiation of naive T cells into Th1 cells or Th17 cells. Interleukin (IL)-17A, IL-17F, and IL-22 are produced by Th17 cells, IFN-γ and tumor TNF-α are produced by Th1 cells. These mediators act on keratinocytes, leading to the activation, proliferation, and production of antimicrobial peptides and proteins (AMPs) or chemokines.

colleagues[82] reported on TNF-α and inducible nitric oxide synthase-producing DCs. These cells have the phenotype of CD1c⁻ and CD11c⁺ DCs. They are also referred to as 6-sulfo LacNAc (slan) DCs by the selective expression of the slan residue on the P-selectin glycoprotein ligand 1 membrane molecule.[83] These inflammatory DCs respond to complexes formed of LL-37 and self-RNA via TLR7 signaling and enable Th1/Th17 cells to produce IL-17, IL-22, TNF-α, and IFN-γ more powerfully than classic CD1c⁺ DCs.[83]

Again, vitamin D is an important keyword in understanding the relationship between psoriasis and cathelicidin. Vitamin D analogs have been used in the topical treatment of psoriasis for a long time. They are known to promote clinical improvement in psoriatic plaques, and have been speculated to act through the stimulation of cellular differentiation and inhibition of proliferation.[84] Recently, there are reports that topical calcipotriol suppresses the expressions of hBD2, hBD3, IL-17A, IL-17F, and IL-8 in psoriatic plaques,[70] and that topically applied 1,25(OH)$_2$D3 induces CD4⁺CD25⁺ regulatory T cells.[85] On the other hand, vitamin D3 is a strong inducer of cathelicidin expression in keratinocytes and monocytes.[25] These results may seem to be paradoxical because LL-37 generally induces inflammation.

However, Dombrowski and colleagues[86] have shown that LL-37 also serves as an anti-inflammatory agent by blocking activation of the DNA-sensing inflammasomes. They also have indicated that intracellular or cytosolic LL-37 blocks the DNA-triggered formation of AIM2 inflammasomes in keratinocytes, inhibiting IL-1β release. Therefore, the location of LL-37 and DNA may be crucial for their proinflammatory or anti-inflammatory effects.[80]

Several studies have focused on the associations between AMPs and other therapies of psoriasis. Peric and colleagues[87] have shown that IL-17A enhances cathelicidin expression induced by vitamin D_3 in keratinocytes. Hegyi and colleagues[88] reported that the expression of S100A7 and S100A15 in psoriatic skin was attenuated after the application of the vitamin D analog calcipotriol. Chamorro and colleagues[89] have described that LL-37 suppresses apoptosis in keratinocytes via a cyclooxygenase-2-dependent mechanism, including inhibitor of apoptosis-2, suggesting that this peptide might contribute to the resistance to apoptosis of dermal endothelial cells in psoriasis. Vahavihu and colleagues[90] reported that narrowband UVB treatment induces cathelicidin expression by correcting vitamin D insufficiency. Also, the decrease or downregulation of LL-37 by cyclosporine A,[91] etanercept, a biologic TNF-α blocker,[92] has been detected. Lin and colleagues[93] stated that there are MCET and neutrophil extracellular traps in psoriatic plaque and they include LL-37.

Atopic Dermatitis

In contrast with rosacea or psoriasis, the induction of some AMPs, such as cathelicidin, hBD2, hBD3, and dermcidin, was found to be lower in AD lesions than expected, despite the presence of skin inflammation.[72,73,94–97] On the other hand, RNase7 and psoriasin are induced in AD lesional skin by barrier disruption.[98] The defective expression of AMPs has been linked to a higher propensity to S aureus colonization, which is known to have an important role in the exacerbation of the infection and is correlated with the extent and severity of atopic skin lesions (Fig. 3).[99] In AD, the proportion of S aureus was greater during disease flares than at baseline or post-treatment and correlated with increased disease severity. Representation of the skin commensal S epidermidis was also significantly increased during flares of AD. Following AD therapy, increases in Streptococcus, Propionibacterium, and Corynebacterium species were observed.[100] Interestingly, there are also some reports about vitamin

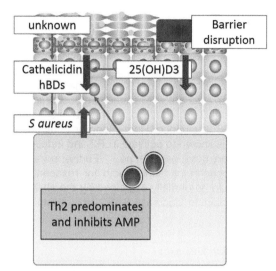

Fig. 3. Atopic dermatitis and AMPs. Under normal conditions barrier disruption will trigger expression of AMPs such as cathelicidin and hBDs. The mechanism for this increase can involve activation of vitamin D or unknown events. In atopic dermatitis the altered T activation and shift in Th2 cytokines leads to suppression of AMP expression and is associated with increased S aureus survival.

D deficiency in AD patients. Kanda and colleagues[96] reported that serum levels of LL-37 and 25(OH)D3 were decreased in patients with AD compared with normal donors. Other reports have suggested that vitamin D deficiency may be related to the severity of AD through inverse correlation between serum levels of 25(OH)D3,[101] or between cord serum level of 25(OH)D3 and risk of transient early wheezing and onset of AD.[102] Also, Samochocki and colleagues[103] reported that the frequency of bacterial skin infections was higher in patients with AD who had lower 25(OH)D3 levels, and that both the mean objective Scoring Atopic Dermatitis (SCORAD) and SCORAD index were lower after the supplementation of vitamin D. Pilot studies have been attempted to compensate for the defective expression of AMPs in the skin of patients suffering from AD by oral vitamin D administration.[30]

Wounds

Dorschner and colleagues[16] demonstrated that AMPs are induced in the skin by injury. LL-37 contributes to cutaneous wound healing by stimulating re-epithelialization.[104] LL-37 also induces neovascularization, which is mediated by formyl peptide receptor-like 1 signaling in endothelial cells, and the cathelicidin-mediated angiogenesis is important for cutaneous wound neovascularization.[41]

Furthermore, LL-37 induces proliferation and migration by human endothelial cells.[105]

Acne Vulgaris

Shibata and colleagues[51] showed that *Propionibacterium acnes* enhanced glucocorticoid-dependent TLR2 induction, which was abolished by RU486, a glucocorticoid receptor antagonist. *P acnes* is known to activate TLR2 and induce inflammatory cytokines in acne.[106] Furthermore, the clinical benefits of retinoic acid for rosacea and acne could be partially explained by the ability of retinoic acid to decrease TLR2 expression and function.[52]

Other Skin Diseases

In systemic lupus erythematosus, the excess presence of LL-37 enables recognition of self-nucleic acids by pDCs.[107] This means that AMPs may exacerbate inflammation and contribute to the disease by permitting autoinflammatory signaling. Actually, several AMPs are also increased in cutaneous lupus erythematosus patients at both gene and protein levels.[108] Expression of AMPs was detected by immunostaining of the skin with viral infectious diseases such as condyloma acuminatum, verruca vulgaris,[109] and molluscum contagiosm.[110] In sexually transmitted diseases, it has been reported that *Herpes simplex* virus (HSV) −2 stimulated epithelial cell production of hBDs and LL-37, and that LL-37 strongly upregulated the expression of human immunodeficiency virus (HIV) receptors in monocyte-derived LCs, thereby enhancing their HIV susceptibility.[111]

SUMMARY

Microbes are a major threat for human health; however, it is not possible to exist without microbes in the environment because they also perform many beneficial functions essential for health. AMPs are naturally occurring antibiotics that have evolved in such a way that they appropriately control the human microbiome and usually resist uncontrolled microbial invasion associated with infection. Unlike the problem of drug resistance seen with pharmaceutically derived antibiotics, AMPs have retained their antimicrobial efficacy versus evolutionary timescales and their composition has changed little. The explanation for the remarkable defense actions of AMPs is that their expression is strictly regulated, and that they are not only antibiotics but also multitalented peptides that are involved in various immunologic responses.

There is much to learn about AMPs. For example, why do humans have only 1 cathelicidin gene, unlike domesticated animals that have many, or the defensin family that includes hundreds of genes? What are the complex regulatory networks that control the expression of AMPs in a cell type and environmental specific manner? How does dysregulation of AMP expression contribute to skin diseases? Are these a critical target for immunotherapy?

Unfortunately, it has historically been difficult to use synthetic AMPs for therapy owing to costs of production, potency, and stability. This may be improving in the near future, and a better understanding of regulatory networks that dictate AMP expression will support strategies to control endogenous production of AMPs during acute infections or during skin diseases. Advances in this field demonstrate the remarkable opportunities AMPs present for improving human health.

REFERENCES

1. Zasloff M. Antimicrobial peptides of multicellular organisms. Nature 2002;415:389–95.
2. Lai Y, Gallo RL. AMPed up immunity: how antimicrobial peptides have multiple roles in immune defense. Trends Immunol 2009;30:131–41.
3. Glaser R, Harder J, Lange H, et al. Antimicrobial psoriasin (S100A7) protects human skin from *Escherichia coli* infection. Nat Immunol 2005;6:57–64.
4. Wimley WC. Describing the mechanism of antimicrobial peptide action with the interfacial activity model. ACS Chem Biol 2010;5:905–17.
5. Mukherjee S, Vaishnava S, Hooper LV. Multilayered regulation of intestinal antimicrobial defense. Cell Mol Life Sci 2008;65:3019–27.
6. Gallo RL, Ono M, Povsic T, et al. Syndecans, cell surface heparan sulfate proteoglycans, are induced by a proline-rich antimicrobial peptide from wounds. Proc Natl Acad Sci U S A 1994;91: 11035–9.
7. Harder J, Bartels J, Christophers E, et al. A peptide antibiotic from human skin. Nature 1997;387:861.
8. Larrick JW, Lee J, Ma S, et al. Structural, functional analysis and localization of the human CAP18 gene. FEBS Lett 1996;398:74–80.
9. Gudmundsson GH, Agerberth B, Odeberg J, et al. The human gene FALL39 and processing of the cathelin precursor to the antibacterial peptide LL-37 in granulocytes. Eur J Biochem 1996;238:325–32.
10. Murakami M, Ohtake T, Dorschner RA, et al. Cathelicidin anti-microbial peptide expression in sweat, an innate defense system for the skin. J Invest Dermatol 2002;119:1090–5.
11. Di Nardo A, Vitiello A, Gallo RL. Cutting edge: mast cell antimicrobial activity is mediated by expression

of cathelicidin antimicrobial peptide. J Immunol 2003;170:2274–8.

12. Wang Z, Lai Y, Bernard JJ, et al. Skin mast cells protect mice against vaccinia virus by triggering mast cell receptor S1PR2 and releasing antimicrobial peptides. J Immunol 2012;188:345–57.

13. von Köckritz-Blickwede M, Goldmann O, Thulin P, et al. Phagocytosis-independent antimicrobial activity of mast cells by means of extracellular trap formation. Blood 2008;111:3070–80.

14. Zhang L-J, Guerrero-Juarez CF, Hata T, et al. Dermal adipocytes protect against invasive *Staphylococcus aureus* skin infection. Science 2015;347: 67–71.

15. Frohm M, Agerberth B, Ahangari G, et al. The expression of the gene coding for the antibacterial peptide LL-37 is induced in human keratinocytes during inflammatory disorders. J Biol Chem 1997; 272:15258–63.

16. Dorschner RA, Pestonjamasp VK, Tamakuwala S, et al. Cutaneous injury induces the release of cathelicidin anti-microbial peptides active against group A Streptococcus. J Invest Dermatol 2001; 117:91–7.

17. Nizet V, Ohtake T, Lauth X, et al. Innate antimicrobial peptide protects the skin from invasive bacterial infection. Nature 2001;414:454–7.

18. Gallo RL, Hooper LV. Epithelial antimicrobial defence of the skin and intestine. Nat Rev Immunol 2012;12:503–16.

19. Grether-Beck S, Felsner I, Brenden H, et al. Urea uptake enhances barrier function and antimicrobial defense in humans by regulating epidermal gene expression. J Invest Dermatol 2012;132:1561–72.

20. Bernard JJ, Cowing-Zitron C, Nakatsuji T, et al. Ultraviolet radiation damages self noncoding RNA and is detected by TLR3. Nat Med 2012;18:1286–90.

21. Sorensen O, Arnljots K, Cowland JB, et al. The human antibacterial cathelicidin, hCAP-18, is synthesized in myelocytes and metamyelocytes and localized to specific granules in neutrophils. Blood 1997;90:2796–803.

22. Yamasaki K, Schauber J, Coda A, et al. Kallikrein-mediated proteolysis regulates the antimicrobial effects of cathelicidins in skin. FASEB J 2006;20: 2068–80.

23. Braff MH, Hawkins MA, Di Nardo A, et al. Structure-function relationships among human cathelicidin peptides: dissociation of antimicrobial properties from host immunostimulatory activities. J Immunol 2005;174:4271–8.

24. Lichtenstein A, Ganz T, Selsted ME, et al. In vitro tumor cell cytolysis mediated by peptide defensins of human and rabbit granulocytes. Blood 1986; 68:1407–10.

25. Wang TT, Nestel FP, Bourdeau V, et al. Cutting edge: 1,25-dihydroxyvitamin D3 is a direct inducer of antimicrobial peptide gene expression. J Immunol 2004;173:2909–12.

26. Gombart AF, Borregaard N, Koeffler HP. Human cathelicidin antimicrobial peptide (CAMP) gene is a direct target of the vitamin D receptor and is strongly up-regulated in myeloid cells by 1,25-dihydroxyvitamin D3. FASEB J 2005;19: 1067–77.

27. Liu PT, Stenger S, Li H, et al. Toll-like receptor triggering of a vitamin D-mediated human antimicrobial response. Science 2006;311:1770–3.

28. Schauber J, Dorschner RA, Coda AB, et al. Injury enhances TLR2 function and antimicrobial peptide expression through a vitamin D-dependent mechanism. J Clin Invest 2007;117:803–11.

29. Dixon BM, Barker T, McKinnon T, et al. Positive correlation between circulating cathelicidin antimicrobial peptide (hCAP18/LL-37) and 25-hydroxyvitamin D levels in healthy adults. BMC Res Notes 2012;5:575.

30. Hata TR, Kotol P, Jackson M, et al. Administration of oral vitamin D induces cathelicidin production in atopic individuals. J Allergy Clin Immunol 2008; 122:829–31.

31. Hong SP, Kim MJ, Jung MY, et al. Biopositive effects of low-dose UVB on epidermis: coordinate upregulation of antimicrobial peptides and permeability barrier reinforcement. J Invest Dermatol 2008;128:2880–7.

32. Tjabringa GS, Aarbiou J, Ninaber DK, et al. The antimicrobial peptide LL-37 activates innate immunity at the airway epithelial surface by transactivation of the epidermal growth factor receptor. J Immunol 2003;171:6690–6.

33. Tokumaru S, Sayama K, Shirakata Y, et al. Induction of keratinocyte migration via transactivation of the epidermal growth factor receptor by the antimicrobial peptide LL-37. J Immunol 2005; 175:4662–8.

34. Schutte BC, McCray PB Jr. β-defensins in lung host defense. Annu Rev Physiol 2002;64:709–48.

35. Cogen AL, Yamasaki K, Sanchez KM, et al. Selective antimicrobial action is provided by phenol-soluble modulins derived from *Staphylococcus epidermidis*, a normal resident of the skin. J Invest Dermatol 2010;130:192–200.

36. Iwase T, Uehara Y, Shinji H, et al. *Staphylococcus epidermidis* Esp inhibits *Staphylococcus aureus* biofilm formation and nasal colonization. Nature 2010;465:346–9.

37. Otto M, Sussmuth R, Vuong C, et al. Inhibition of virulence factor expression in *Staphylococcus aureus* by the *Staphylococcus epidermidis* agr pheromone and derivatives. FEBS Lett 1999;450:257–62.

38. Crawford GH, Pelle MT, James WD. Rosacea: I. Etiology, pathogenesis, and subtype classification. J Am Acad Dermatol 2004;51:327–41.

39. Takeda K, Kaisho T, Akira S. Toll-like receptors. Annu Rev Immunol 2003;21:335–76.

40. Meylan E, Tschopp J, Karin M. Intracellular pattern recognition receptors in the host response. Nature 2006;442:39–44.

41. Koczulla R, von Degenfeld G, Kupatt C, et al. An angiogenic role for the human peptide antibiotic LL-37/hCAP-18. J Clin Invest 2003;111:1665–72.

42. Yamasaki K, Di Nardo A, Bardan A, et al. Increased serine protease activity and cathelicidin promotes skin inflammation in rosacea. Nat Med 2007;13:975–80.

43. De Y, Chen Q, Schmidt AP, et al. LL-37, the neutrophil granule- and epithelial cell-derived cathelicidin, utilizes formyl peptide receptor-like 1 (FPRL1) as a receptor to chemoattract human peripheral blood neutrophils, monocytes, and T cells. J Exp Med 2000;192:1069–74.

44. Murakami M, Lopez-Garcia B, Braff M, et al. Postsecretory processing generates multiple cathelicidins for enhanced topical antimicrobial defense. J Immunol 2004;172:3070–7.

45. Detmar M, Brown LF, Claffey KP, et al. Overexpression of vascular permeability factor/vascular endothelial growth factor and its receptors in psoriasis. J Exp Med 1994;180:1141–6.

46. Chen CJ, Kono H, Golenbock D, et al. Identification of a key pathway required for the sterile inflammatory response triggered by dying cells. Nat Med 2007;13:851–6.

47. Taylor KR, Yamasaki K, Radek KA, et al. Recognition of hyaluronan released in sterile injury involves a unique receptor complex dependent on Toll-like receptor 4, CD44, and MD-2. J Biol Chem 2007;282:18265–75.

48. Yamasaki K, Kanada K, Macleod DT, et al. TLR2 expression is increased in rosacea and stimulates enhanced serine protease production by keratinocytes. J Invest Dermatol 2011;131:688–97.

49. Schauber J, Dorschner RA, Yamasaki K, et al. Control of the innate epithelial antimicrobial response is cell-type specific and dependent on relevant microenvironmental stimuli. Immunology 2006;118:509–19.

50. Morizane S, Yamasaki K, Kabigting FD, et al. Kallikrein expression and cathelicidin processing are independently controlled in keratinocytes by calcium, vitamin D3, and retinoic acid. J Invest Dermatol 2010;130:1297–306.

51. Shibata M, Katsuyama M, Onodera T, et al. Glucocorticoids enhance Toll-like receptor 2 expression in human keratinocytes stimulated with *Propionibacterium acnes* or proinflammatory cytokines. J Invest Dermatol 2009;129:375–82.

52. Liu PT, Krutzik SR, Kim J, et al. Cutting edge: all-trans retinoic acid down-regulates TLR2 expression and function. J Immunol 2005;174:2467–70.

53. Dispenza MC, Wolpert EB, Gilliland KL, et al. Systemic isotretinoin therapy normalizes exaggerated TLR-2-mediated innate immune responses in acne patients. J Invest Dermatol 2012;132:2198–205.

54. Coda AB, Hata T, Miller J, et al. Cathelicidin, kallikrein 5, and serine protease activity is inhibited during treatment of rosacea with azelaic acid 15% gel. J Am Acad Dermatol 2013;69:570–7.

55. Kanada KN, Nakatsuji T, Gallo RL. Doxycycline indirectly inhibits proteolytic activation of tryptic kallikrein-related peptidases and activation of cathelicidin. J Invest Dermatol 2012;132:1435–42.

56. Muto Y, Wang Z, Vanderberghe M, et al. Mast cells are key mediators of cathelicidin-initiated skin inflammation in rosacea. J Invest Dermatol 2014;134:2728–36.

57. Two AM, Hata TR, Nakatsuji T, et al. Reduction in serine protease activity correlates with improved rosacea severity in a small, randomized pilot study of a topical serine protease inhibitor. J Invest Dermatol 2014;134:1143–5.

58. Nestle FO, Kaplan DH, Barker J. Psoriasis. N Engl J Med 2009;361:496–509.

59. Albanesi C, De Pita O, Girolomoni G. Resident skin cells in psoriasis: a special look at the pathogenetic functions of keratinocytes. Clin Dermatol 2007;25:581–8.

60. Buchau AS, Gallo RL. Innate immunity and antimicrobial defense systems in psoriasis. Clin Dermatol 2007;25:616–24.

61. Harder J, Schroder JM. Psoriatic scales: a promising source for the isolation of human skin-derived antimicrobial proteins. J Leukoc Biol 2005;77:476–86.

62. Harder J, Bartels J, Christophers E, et al. Isolation and characterization of human beta -defensin-3, a novel human inducible peptide antibiotic. J Biol Chem 2001;276:5707–13.

63. Hollox EJ, Huffmeier U, Zeeuwen PL, et al. Psoriasis is associated with increased beta-defensin genomic copy number. Nat Genet 2008;40:23–5.

64. Nomura I, Goleva E, Howell MD, et al. Cytokine milieu of atopic dermatitis, as compared to psoriasis, skin prevents induction of innate immune response genes. J Immunol 2003;171:3262–9.

65. Liang SC, Tan XY, Luxenberg DP, et al. Interleukin (IL)-22 and IL-17 are coexpressed by Th17 cells and cooperatively enhance expression of antimicrobial peptides. J Exp Med 2006;203:2271–9.

66. Lande R, Chamilos G, Ganguly D, et al. Cationic antimicrobial peptides in psoriatic skin cooperate to break innate tolerance to self-DNA. Eur J Immunol 2015;45:203–13.

67. Madsen P, Rasmussen HH, Leffers H, et al. Molecular cloning, occurrence, and expression of a novel partially secreted protein "psoriasin" that is highly

up-regulated in psoriatic skin. J Invest Dermatol 1991;97:701–12.

68. Eckert RL, Broome AM, Ruse M, et al. S100 proteins in the epidermis. J Invest Dermatol 2004; 123:23–33.

69. Glaser R, Meyer-Hoffert U, Harder J, et al. The antimicrobial protein psoriasin (S100A7) is upregulated in atopic dermatitis and after experimental skin barrier disruption. J Invest Dermatol 2009; 129:641–9.

70. Peric M, Koglin S, Dombrowski Y, et al. Vitamin D analogs differentially control antimicrobial peptide/"alarmin" expression in psoriasis. PLoS One 2009;4:e6340.

71. Jinquan T, Vorum H, Larsen CG, et al. Psoriasin: a novel chemotactic protein. J Invest Dermatol 1996; 107:5–10.

72. Ong PY, Ohtake T, Brandt C, et al. Endogenous antimicrobial peptides and skin infections in atopic dermatitis. N Engl J Med 2002;347:1151–60.

73. Lande R, Gregorio J, Facchinetti V, et al. Plasmacytoid dendritic cells sense self-DNA coupled with antimicrobial peptide. Nature 2007;449:564–9.

74. Hemmi H, Takeuchi O, Kawai T, et al. A Toll-like receptor recognizes bacterial DNA. Nature 2000; 408:740–5.

75. Funk J, Langeland T, Schrumpf E, et al. Psoriasis induced by interferon-alpha. Br J Dermatol 1991; 125:463–5.

76. Hida S, Ogasawara K, Sato K, et al. CD8(+) T cell-mediated skin disease in mice lacking IRF-2, the transcriptional attenuator of interferon-alpha/beta signaling. Immunity 2000;13:643–55.

77. Suomela S, Cao L, Bowcock A, et al. Interferon alpha-inducible protein 27 (IFI27) is upregulated in psoriatic skin and certain epithelial cancers. J Invest Dermatol 2004;122:717–21.

78. Banchereau J, Pascual V, Palucka AK. Autoimmunity through cytokine-induced dendritic cell activation. Immunity 2004;20:539–50.

79. Nestle FO, Conrad C, Tun-Kyi A, et al. Plasmacytoid predendritic cells initiate psoriasis through interferon-alpha production. J Exp Med 2005;202: 135–43.

80. Morizane S, Yamasaki K, Muhleisen B, et al. Cathelicidin antimicrobial peptide LL-37 in psoriasis enables keratinocyte reactivity against TLR9 ligands. J Invest Dermatol 2012;132:135–43.

81. Ganguly D, Chamilos G, Lande R, et al. Self-RNA-antimicrobial peptide complexes activate human dendritic cells through TLR7 and TLR8. J Exp Med 2009;206:1983–94.

82. Lowes MA, Chamian F, Abello MV, et al. Increase in TNF-α and inducible nitric oxide synthase-expressing dendritic cells in psoriasis and reduction with efalizumab (anti-CD11a). Proc Natl Acad Sci U S A 2005;102:19057–62.

83. Hansel A, Gunther C, Ingwersen J, et al. Human slan (6-sulfo LacNAc) dendritic cells are inflammatory dermal dendritic cells in psoriasis and drive strong TH17/TH1 T-cell responses. J Allergy Clin Immunol 2011;127:787–94.e1-9.

84. Fogh K, Kragballe K. Recent developments in vitamin D analogs. Curr Pharm Des 2000;6: 961–72.

85. Gorman S, Kuritzky LA, Judge MA, et al. Topically applied 1,25-dihydroxyvitamin D3 enhances the suppressive activity of CD4+CD25+ cells in the draining lymph nodes. J Immunol 2007;179: 6273–83.

86. Dombrowski Y, Peric M, Koglin S, et al. Cytosolic DNA triggers inflammasome activation in keratinocytes in psoriatic lesions. Sci Transl Med 2011;3: 82ra38.

87. Peric M, Koglin S, Kim SM, et al. IL-17A enhances vitamin D3-induced expression of cathelicidin antimicrobial peptide in human keratinocytes. J Immunol 2008;181:8504–12.

88. Hegyi Z, Zwicker S, Bureik D, et al. Vitamin D analog calcipotriol suppresses the Th17 cytokine–induced proinflammatory S100 "alarmins" psoriasin (S100A7) and koebnerisin (S100A15) in psoriasis. J Invest Dermatol 2012;132:1416–24.

89. Chamorro CI, Weber G, Gronberg A, et al. The human antimicrobial peptide LL-37 suppresses apoptosis in keratinocytes. J Invest Dermatol 2009;129:937–44.

90. Vahavihu K, Ala-Houhala M, Peric M, et al. Narrowband ultraviolet B treatment improves vitamin D balance and alters antimicrobial peptide expression in skin lesions of psoriasis and atopic dermatitis. Br J Dermatol 2010;163:321–8.

91. Kanda N, Ishikawa T, Kamata M, et al. Increased serum leucine, leucine-37 levels in psoriasis: positive and negative feedback loops of leucine, leucine-37 and pro- or anti-inflammatory cytokines. Hum Immunol 2010;71:1161–71.

92. Gambichler T, Kobus S, Kobus A, et al. Expression of antimicrobial peptides and proteins in etanercept-treated psoriasis patients. Regul Pept 2011;167:163–6.

93. Lin AM, Rubin CJ, Khandpur R, et al. Mast cells and neutrophils release IL-17 through extracellular trap formation in psoriasis. J Immunol 2011;187: 490–500.

94. Hata TR, Kotol P, Boguniewicz M, et al. History of eczema herpeticum is associated with the inability to induce human beta-defensin (HBD)-2, HBD-3 and cathelicidin in the skin of patients with atopic dermatitis. Br J Dermatol 2010;163:659–61.

95. Mallbris L, Carlen L, Wei T, et al. Injury downregulates the expression of the human cathelicidin protein hCAP18/LL-37 in atopic dermatitis. Exp Dermatol 2010;19:442–9.

96. Kanda N, Hau CS, Tada Y, et al. Decreased serum LL-37 and vitamin D3 levels in atopic dermatitis: relationship between IL-31 and oncostatin M. Allergy 2012;67:804–12.

97. Rieg S, Steffen H, Seeber S, et al. Deficiency of dermcidin-derived antimicrobial peptides in sweat of patients with atopic dermatitis correlates with an impaired innate defense of human skin in vivo. J Immunol 2005;174:8003–10.

98. Harder J, Dressel S, Wittersheim M, et al. Enhanced expression and secretion of antimicrobial peptides in atopic dermatitis and after superficial skin injury. J Invest Dermatol 2010;130:1355–64.

99. Miller LS, Sorensen OE, Liu PT, et al. TGF-alpha regulates TLR expression and function on epidermal keratinocytes. J Immunol 2005;174:6137–43.

100. Kong HH, Oh J, Deming C, et al. Temporal shifts in the skin microbiome associated with disease flares and treatment in children with atopic dermatitis. Genome Res 2012;22:850–9.

101. Peroni DG, Piacentini GL, Cametti E, et al. Correlation between serum 25-hydroxyvitamin D levels and severity of atopic dermatitis in children. Br J Dermatol 2011;164:1078–82.

102. Baïz N, Dargent-Molina P, Wark JD, et al. Cord serum 25-hydroxyvitamin D and risk of early childhood transient wheezing and atopic dermatitis. J Allergy Clin Immunol 2014;133:147–53.

103. Samochocki Z, Bogaczewicz J, Jeziorkowska R, et al. Vitamin D effects in atopic dermatitis. J Am Acad Dermatol 2013;69:238–44.

104. Heilborn JD, Nilsson MF, Kratz G, et al. The cathelicidin anti-microbial peptide LL-37 is involved in re-epithelialization of human skin wounds and is lacking in chronic ulcer epithelium. J Invest Dermatol 2003;120:379–89.

105. Ramos R, Silva JP, Rodrigues AC, et al. Wound healing activity of the human antimicrobial peptide LL37. Peptides 2011;32:1469–76.

106. Kim J, Ochoa MT, Krutzik SR, et al. Activation of toll-like receptor 2 in acne triggers inflammatory cytokine responses. J Immunol 2002;169:1535–41.

107. Lande R, Ganguly D, Facchinetti V, et al. Neutrophils activate plasmacytoid dendritic cells by releasing self-DNA-peptide complexes in systemic lupus erythematosus. Sci Transl Med 2011;3:73ra19.

108. Kreuter A, Jaouhar M, Skrygan M, et al. Expression of antimicrobial peptides in different subtypes of cutaneous lupus erythematosus. J Am Acad Dermatol 2011;65:125–33.

109. Conner K, Nern K, Rudisill J, et al. The antimicrobial peptide LL-37 is expressed by keratinocytes in condyloma acuminatum and verruca vulgaris. J Am Acad Dermatol 2002;47:347–50.

110. Meyer-Hoffert U, Schwarz T, Schroder JM, et al. Increased expression of human beta-defensin 3 in mollusca contagiosum. Clin Exp Dermatol 2010;35:190–2.

111. Ogawa Y, Kawamura T, Matsuzawa T, et al. Antimicrobial peptide LL-37 produced by HSV-2-infected keratinocytes enhances HIV infection of Langerhans cells. Cell Host Microbe 2013;13:77–86.

Mosaic Disorders of the PI3K/PTEN/AKT/TSC/mTORC1 Signaling Pathway

CrossMark

Neera Nathan, MD[a], Kim M. Keppler-Noreuil, MD[b],
Leslie G. Biesecker, MD[b], Joel Moss, MD, PhD[c],
Thomas N. Darling, MD, PhD[a],*

KEYWORDS

- Mosaicism • mTORC1 • PIK3CA-related overgrowth spectrum • Proteus syndrome
- Tuberous sclerosis complex • PTEN hamartoma tumor syndrome • Next-generation sequencing
- Sirolimus

KEY POINTS

- Mosaicism may be considered in sporadic cases; there should be a negative history in ancestral generations or siblings but offspring may be affected through gonadal mosaicism.
- A patchy distribution of cutaneous features and tissue overgrowth or disseminated disease that is mild should raise suspicion for mosaicism.
- Next-generation sequencing, or other methods for detecting low frequency alleles, of affected tissue is frequently necessary to identify the genetic basis of mosaic conditions.
- Drugs that target proteins along the PI3K/PTEN/AKT/TSC/mTORC1 signaling pathway have shown promise in the treatment of these disorders.

INTRODUCTION

Mosaicism may occur as a somatic mutation occurring during embryogenesis, resulting in an organism composed of 2 (or more) genetically distinct cell lineages.[1] The resulting phenotype depends on the numbers and organization of abnormal cells in relation to normal cells and how the mutation affects cellular function.[2,3] When the mutation affects cell signaling pathways regulating cell growth, apoptosis, or migration, dramatic regional alterations in the appearance of the skin can occur sometimes with regional overgrowth or tumor susceptibility. Dermatologists are frequent observers of these mosaic conditions and play important roles in diagnosis and management.

Somatic mutations in any of the genes in the PI3K/PTEN/AKT/TSC/mTORC1 signaling pathway (**Fig. 1**) may result in a spectrum of abnormal growth, ranging from an isolated small skin lesion

Funding or Support: Dr J. Moss was supported by the Intramural Research Program, National Institutes of Health, National Heart, Lung, and Blood Institute. Dr L.G. Biesecker and Dr K.M. Keppler-Noreuil were supported by the Intramural Research Program of the National Human Genome Research Institute. Dr T.N. Darling was supported by National Institutes of Health R01 AR062080. This research was also made possible through a Doris Duke Charitable Foundation Clinical Research Mentorship grant (#2014088).
Conflicts of Interest Disclosures: None reported.
^a Department of Dermatology, Uniformed Services University of the Health Sciences, 4301 Jones Bridge Road, Bethesda, MD 20814, USA; ^b Medical Genomics and Metabolic Genetics Branch, National Human Genome Research Institute, Building 49, Room 4A56, 49 Convent Drive, National Institutes of Health, Bethesda, MD 20892, USA; ^c Cardiovascular and Pulmonary Branch, National Heart, Lung, and Blood Institute, Building 10, Room 6D05, 10 Center Drive, National Institutes of Health, Bethesda, MD 20892-1590, USA
* Corresponding author.
E-mail address: thomas.darling@usuhs.edu

derm.theclinics.com

with minimal or no overgrowth to extensive skin involvement with striking extremity enlargement and tumor susceptibility.[4–7] Proteus syndrome, caused by mutations in *AKT1*, and the *PIK3CA*-related overgrowth spectrum (PROS) may be considered archetypal mosaic disorders, given the patchy distribution of disease features.[8,9] Tuberous sclerosis complex (TSC), caused by mutations in either *TSC1* or *TSC2*, and *PTEN* hamartoma tumor syndrome (PHTS) are most frequently associated with germline mutations, but mosaic forms also appear as isolated (simplex or sporadic) occurrences.[10–12] This article primarily focuses on these entities, chosen for their shared abnormalities in a signaling pathway and analogous or overlapping phenotypes.

PI3K/PTEN/AKT/TSC/MTORC1 SIGNALING PATHWAY AND OVERGROWTH

Cell growth is mediated by extracellular cues and may occur via increasing cell mass or cell division

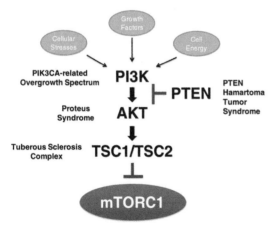

Fig. 1. Disorders of the mTORC1 signaling pathway.

or by suppression of apoptosis. Mechanistic target of rapamycin (mTOR) complex 1 (mTORC1) is a central regulator of cell growth[13] that is disrupted in many human disorders of cell proliferation, including cancers.[4,5,13–15] Under normal conditions, mTORC1 is sensitive to inputs from diverse cellular and environmental cues (see **Fig. 1**), including the phosphoinositide-3-kinase (PI3K) pathway. In short, growth factors stimulate PI3K, which then converts phosphatidylinositol (4,5)-bisphosphate (PIP2) to phosphatidylinositol (3,4,5)-trisphosphate (PIP3) and permits activation of AKT. PTEN dephosphorylates PIP3 to PIP2, thereby exerting inhibitory control on AKT.[16] AKT phosphorylates several proteins, including the TSC1-TSC2 complex, and thus alleviates negative control on mTOR to promote cell growth (see **Fig. 1**).

PTEN, *TSC1*, and *TSC2* are tumor suppressors. For each of these genes, a germline mutation causes a loss of function allele, leading to a syndrome with susceptibility to multiple tumors. Tumorigenesis involves inactivation of the second allele, typically via a second-hit somatic mutation in the wild-type allele.[6,16] Loss of function of *PTEN* results in increased levels of PIP3 and alleviates inhibitory control on AKT to cause tumor formation in PHTS.[17] Biallelic mutations in *TSC1* or *TSC2* result in increased Ras homolog enriched in brain (Rheb)-GTP, which activates signaling through mTORC1, causing tumor formation in TSC.[18] Although the PHTS and TSC are typically caused by germline mutations, both can have mosaic presentations, often with mild disease or later onset than inherited disease.[11,19–23]

PIK3CA, a gene encoding the catalytic subunit of PI3K, and *AKT1* are oncogenes and thus a gain of function, or activating mutation in only one copy of the allele is the mechanism of disease.[24,25] Strongly activating mutations in these genes may only be seen in patients through mosaicism.[26,27] Point mutations activating *PIK3CA* have been documented in a variety of mosaic disorders captured under the umbrella term PROS.[9,27] The mosaic presence of an activating mutation in *AKT1* results in Proteus syndrome.[26,28]

PHENOTYPE OF DISORDERS OF THE PI3K/PTEN/AKT/TSC/MTORC1 SIGNALING PATHWAY
Mosaic-Only Oncogenes

It is widely regarded that strongly activating germline mutations in *AKT1* and *PIK3CA* are lethal, with few reported exceptions.[9,26,29] Mutations in these genes result in distinctive segmental, or asymmetric overgrowth syndromes that can involve the bone, muscle, adipose tissue, skin, and/or nerves and may be relatively stable (*PIK3CA*) or progressive (*AKT1* or *PIK3CA*) in course.[9,26,30–32] The severity of the overgrowth may range from a slightly enlarged digit to a gigantic limb.[33,34] Hamartomas, or benign, focal overgrowths resembling their tissue of origin, may also be present.[35] The epidermal nevus and vascular malformation in these disorders (**Fig.** 2A, B) are examples of the Blaschkoid and checkerboard patterns of cutaneous mosaicism, respectively.[36]

Somatic activation in *AKT1* has been linked to Proteus syndrome, an extraordinarily rare disorder (incidence is <1 case per 10 million) that is characterized by sporadic occurrence, asymmetric distribution of lesions, and progressive course.[26,37] Frequent dermatologic lesions include cerebriform connective tissue nevi, lipomas, linear keratinocytic epidermal nevus, and lymphovascular malformations.[8]

PROS represents a broad constellation of somatic disorders caused by activating mutations in *PIK3CA*, including congenital lipomatous overgrowth, vascular malformations, linear keratinocytic epidermal nevi, and skeletal or spinal anomalies (CLOVES) syndrome; fibroadipose hyperplasia or overgrowth; hemihyperplasia multiple lipomatosis; certain megalencephaly syndromes; isolated macrodactyly; isolated lymphatic malformations; seborrheic keratoses; and benign lichenoid keratoses.[30,38,39] The phenotype of this spectrum ranges from isolated disease, such as macrodactyly, megalencephaly, or vascular malformations, to syndromes defined by tissue overgrowth, vascular malformations, and epidermal nevi.[9,30,40,41] Because several individuals with Klippel-Trenaunay syndrome (KTS), which bears clinical semblance to PROS, have pathogenic *PIK3CA* mutations, KTS may be under the PROS umbrella.[42]

Germline or Mosaic Tumor Suppressor Genes

PHTS represents a spectrum of diseases caused by mutations in the PTEN tumor suppressor gene, including Cowden syndrome and Bannayan-Riley-Ruvalcaba syndrome (BRRS).[43] Cowden syndrome is an autosomal-dominant condition characterized by skin hamartomas and mixed benign and malignant tumors of the thyroid, breast, and endometrium.[44] Characteristic mucocutaneous lesions include trichilemmomas, acral keratoses, and oral papillomatosis, and are usually present by the third decade.[10,44] Malignancy risk is greatest for breast cancer (approximately 85%) and is increased for thyroid cancer, endometrial cancer, colon cancer, and melanoma.[43]

BRRS is usually congenital in onset and cutaneous manifestations include pigmented macules of the glans penis,[45] although formal diagnostic criteria have not yet been defined.[43] Given the clinical overlap and known allelism of BRRS and

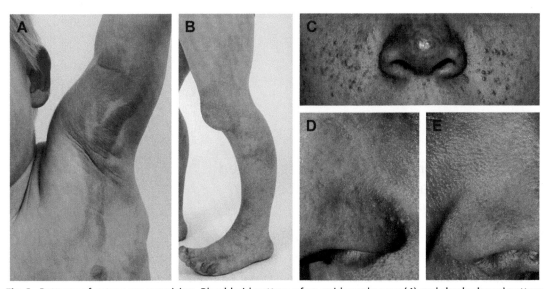

Fig. 2. Patterns of cutaneous mosaicism. Blaschkoid pattern of an epidermal nevus (*A*) and checkerboard pattern of a capillary malformation (*B*) in children with Proteus syndrome. Disseminated (*C*) and type 1 segmental mosaicism (*D, E*) in women with tuberous sclerosis complex. Angiofibromas are observed in the left nasal groove (*D*) but absent from the right in the same individual (*E*). Written informed consent for patients included in this figure was obtained according to NIH protocols 00-H-0051, 95-H-0186, and/or 82-H-0032 (*C–E*).

Cowden syndrome, some assert that they are 1 condition with distinct manifestations in childhood and adulthood, respectively.[46]

For conditions with autosomal-dominant inheritance, 3 categories of mosaicism exist (**Fig. 3**).[3] Disseminated mosaicism is perhaps the most common; the phenotype is usually clinically similar to germline disease with multiple lesions and/or tumors.[1,36,47] Segmental mosaicism may be categorized based on the genetic background of the organism. Type 1 segmental mosaicism describes a localized postzygotic heterozygous mutation in an organism with 2 otherwise normal alleles, resulting in expected disease manifestations restricted to a discrete region. Type 2 segmental mosaicism describes an organism with a localized postzygotic mutation in *trans* (ie, on the otherwise

normal allele) to a mutant allele that was inherited from a heterozygous parent, resulting in biallelic mutations in some cell lines. If the heterozygous mutant state causes disease, as in TSC or PHTS, then type 2 segmental mosaicism results in a clinical phenotype with a more severe segment of disease in a patient with otherwise typical disease distribution.[1,36,47–49]

Mosaicism has been genetically confirmed in several cases among the 10% to 40% of patients with de novo mutations in *PTEN*.[10] Most reports describe disseminated mosaicism, resulting in an anatomically diffuse distribution of cutaneous hamartomas and mixed internal lesions that are clinically difficult to distinguish from inherited or de novo, nonmosaic Cowden syndrome disease.[19,20,50] Interestingly, there have also

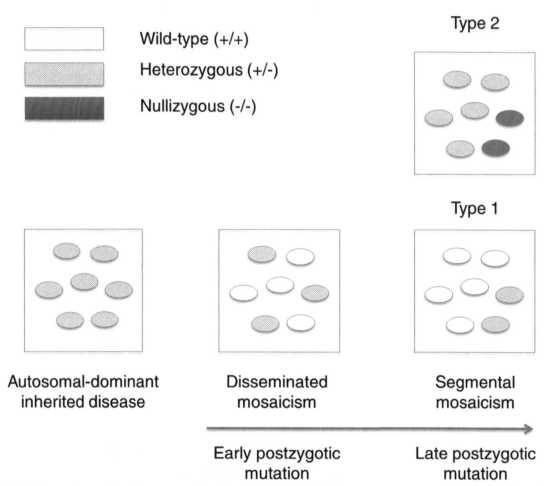

Fig. 3. Types of mosaicism in autosomal dominant conditions. Each square represents an individual and ovals represent cells. In disseminated mosaicism, a postzygotic mutation occurs relatively early in development so that mutant cells are scattered among normal cells throughout the body. In type 1 segmental mosaicism, a postzygotic mutation occurs that is limited to certain body regions. In type 2 segmental mosaicism, the individual inherits only 1 functional copy of the gene and, late in embryogenesis, a postzygotic mutation occurs, resulting in a region that is nullizygous with accentuated disease.

been isolated occurrences of patients with germline *PTEN* mutations that harbor loss of *PTEN* heterozygosity in lesions not characteristic of Cowden syndrome or BRRS.[22,51] Because of its distinct clinical picture, type 2 segmental mosaicism for *PTEN* was termed segmental overgrowth, lipomatosis, arteriovenous malformations, and epidermal nevi (SOLAMEN) syndrome to reflect the presence of these features in addition to those consistent with a germline *PTEN* mutation.[22,46] Similarly, an overgrowth of fat, blood vessels, and fibrous tissue (termed the PTEN hamartoma of soft tissue) has been described in individuals with Cowden syndrome and BRRS,[52] although type 2 segmental mosaicism of the *PTEN* gene has not been molecularly confirmed in these lesions.

TSC is a neurocutaneous syndrome inherited in an autosomal-dominant pattern characterized by hamartomas in multiple organ systems, including the brain, kidneys, lungs, and skin.[53,54] Hypomelanotic macules, angiofibromas, shagreen patches, ungual fibromas, and fibrous cephalic plaques are among the most frequent and specific cutaneous findings.[55–57] Oral findings include oral fibromas and dental enamel pits.[57,58] Noninvasive, visceral hamartomas can be harmful due to hemorrhage risk or impingement on adjacent structures.[12] A subset of TSC patients have no mutation identified using conventional analysis and many of these patients are mosaic.[11] A postzygotic mutation in *TSC1* or *TSC2* before neural crest cell differentiation may explain disseminated TSC-related skin lesions, including bilateral angiofibromas (Fig. 2C), ungual fibromas, and hypomelanotic macules.[11,59–62] Unilateral facial angiofibromas are suspected to represent type 1 segmental mosaicism (Fig. 2D, E).[63]

COMPARING PHENOTYPES

Although these disorders are distinctive, there is overlap in the phenotypes associated with

mutations of *PIK3CA*, *PTEN*, *TSC1*, *TSC2*, and *AKT1*, which may be expected given their common pathway and mosaic pathogenesis. Disorders of this axis may be broadly characterized by frequency of 1 or more of the following features: segmental overgrowth, hamartomas, or malignant tumors (Table 1). Because all 4 conditions are characterized by hamartomas, Table 2 contrasts the specific types of hamartomas observed in these conditions.

Proteus syndrome and PROS may be difficult to clinically distinguish; however, stable course and/or lack of cerebriform connective tissue nevus may point toward a PROS diagnosis.[9] Type 2 segmental Cowden syndrome may also resemble Proteus syndrome or PROS but can be identified by presence of orofacial papules and/or hamartomas of the thyroid, breast, and endometrium.[22]

PROPOSED MECHANISMS OF PHENOTYPE DIVERGENCE
Timing of Mutations

Variation in the timing of postzygotic mutations may cause phenotypic variability, conferring a spectrum of disease burden. In TSC and PHTS, individuals with an early postzygotic mutation often have similar disease features and distribution of disease to those with a germline mutation.[19,20,50,59] More specifically, postzygotic mutations occurring before or after cell differentiation events may explain certain disease presentations. For example, a *TSC2* mutation occurring during neuroectodermal development may explain the presence of tubers in TSC but the absence of subependymal nodules,[64] whereas a mutation in neural crest cells after migration from the neural tube may account for complete absence of neuroanatomical brain involvement in these patients.[65] A *PIK3CA* mutation that occurs before germ layer differentiation may manifest as multisystem disease in PROS with cortical abnormalities (ectodermal origin) and capillary malformations

---

Table 1
Types of abnormal growth observed with mosaic mutations of the PI3K/PTEN/AKT/TSC/mTORC1 signaling pathway

	PIK3CA	PTEN	AKT1	TSC1/TSC2
	PROS	PHTS	Proteus Syndrome	Tuberous Sclerosis Complex
Segmental Overgrowth	***	*	***	*
Hamartomas	***	***	***	***
Malignant Tumors	*	***	*	*

Abbreviations: ***, common; *, uncommon; PHTS, PTEN hamartoma tumor syndrome; PROS, *PIK3CA*-related overgrowth spectrum.

Table 2
Mucocutaneous hamartomas of mosaic disorders of the PI3K/PTEN/AKT/TSC/mTORC1 signaling pathway

	PIK3CA	PTEN	AKT1	TSC1/TSC2
	PROS	PHTS	Proteus Syndrome	TSC
Facial Papules	—	***	—	***
Epidermal Nevus	***	*	***	*
Connective Tissue Nevus	*	*	***	***
Cutaneous Vascular malformation	***	*	***	*
Oral Papules	—	***	—	***

Abbreviations: ***, common; *, uncommon; PHTS, PTEN hamartoma tumor syndrome; PROS, *PIK3CA*-related overgrowth spectrum.

(mesodermal origin).[30] In contrast, a localized postzygotic mutation will produce disease manifestations restricted to tissue type and/or a segment of the body, as demonstrated in a case of Proteus syndrome with only bilateral cerebriform connective tissue nevus and lower extremity varicose veins.[66]

Tissue Specificity

In addition to timing of mutation, tissue type in which the mosaic mutation resides seems to influence the clinical presentation; for instance, an activating *AKT1* mutation in keratinocytes is responsible for epidermal nevus formation, yet the same mutation in fibroblasts produces an entirely different clinical entity (ie, the cerebriform connective tissue nevus).[67] In some cases, mutation in a cell restricted to a certain germ layer may additionally affect tissues from a separate layer through cell signaling. Indeed, fibroblast-like cells in TSC-related hamartomas have been shown to release paracrine factors that affect the overlying epidermis.[68]

DIAGNOSIS OF MOSAICISM

Clinical diagnosis alone is often difficult for these conditions, given substantial overlap of characteristic features. Although traditional genetic analysis of mosaic patients can be equally difficult, sampling the affected tissue, rather than blood, using deep sequencing methods seems to have greater diagnostic accuracy.[11,19,22,66,67,69,70] For instance, studies suggest that up to 15% of patients with TSC may be mosaic; however, conventional sequencing methods may fail to detect low levels of the mutant allele in the blood.[11,59–61,71] Next-generation sequencing techniques that analyze angiofibroma samples for genetic mutations are promising to close the diagnostic gap for patients

with no mutation identified from blood samples.[11,69] A similar approach has been used by harvesting epidermal nevi, vascular malformations or overgrown muscle samples to allow molecular diagnosis in patients with Proteus syndrome and PROS.[26,30,40,67,70,72] Mutational analysis of resected dysplastic cerebellar tissue in Cowden syndrome has also been used for mosaic diagnosis.[19] Because all of the conditions discussed here present with at least some pathogenic skin findings, sequencing of DNA isolated from cutaneous tissue samples may be the least invasive, yet effective, way of arriving at molecular diagnosis for these patients.

Although genetic testing may be helpful to guide patient management, caution should be taken when interpreting results. Thus far, the frequency of mutant cells in affected or normal tissue does not accurately correlate with disease burden in disorders of this pathway.[9,20,67,69]

COUNSELING FOR PROGNOSIS AND MANAGEMENT

The presence of seemingly benign skin findings or highly limited disease involvement may have greater clinical importance than is apparent. This example has been recently demonstrated in TSC, in which patients with mild clinically apparent disease in fact harbored serious internal manifestations that caused morbidity and, sometimes, mortality.[12,73] Thus, lifetime surveillance for brain, pulmonary and renal hamartomas is necessary for all patients with TSC, including those with mosaic mutations.[74] Although rare, malignant transformation of benign tumors in TSC has reported.[75] In patients with PHTS, characteristic cutaneous hamartomas may signal the presence of, or impending risk for, internal malignancies. Thus, patients with mosaic and germline PTEN mutations should be routinely monitored for breast, endometrial and thyroid cancers according to current guidelines because even patients with a low frequency of mutant cells may have increased cancer risk.[19,44]

There have been reports of nephroblastomatosis (a premalignant lesion) and Wilms tumor in several patients with PROS and hemihyperplasia.[9,27,40,76] Based on literature citing a 3.3% to 6% risk of tumorigenesis for embryonal tumors in isolated hemihyperplasia, there may be a similar risk for patients with PROS.[76–78] Thus, preliminary recommendations for surveillance have been proposed, including serial ultrasounds of the abdomen but further data are needed to confirm prevalence of tumorigenesis.[30] Although the risk of malignancy in Proteus syndrome and PROS is unknown, the risk of thrombosis and subsequent pulmonary embolism is substantial for patients with Proteus syndrome and PROS. This seems to be most threatening when patients undergo surgery and surgeons need to be aware of this risk. Patient education regarding symptoms suggestive of a thromboembolism is also important.[9,37]

In addition to disease surveillance, reproductive counseling for patients with mosaic disorders warrants special mention. For patients with mosaicism for *TSC1*, *TSC2*, or *PTEN*, mosaic cells may be present in the gonads. Thus, a patient with limited mosaic disease involvement could give birth to a severely affected (nonmosaic) child.[1] The chance that an offspring of a mosaic individual would be affected is difficult to estimate and such patients should be referred for genetic counseling. On the other hand, gonadal mosaicism for a mutation in either *AKT1* or *PIK3CA* is not likely to result in a viable fetus.[26,79]

SUMMARY

The mosaic disorders of the PI3K/PTEN/AKT/TSC/mTORC1 signaling pathway share a common axis but distinct mutations in this pathway are associated with highly variable clinical presentations that are recognizable. These clinical presentations should be genetically confirmed because each condition has unique implications for disease management. This common pathway may provide insight into treatment. For instance, oral mTORC1 inhibitors have shown to reduce the disease burden in TSC,[74,80] have shown promise for vascular malformations and PHTS,[74,81,82] and are currently being investigated for PROS. In vitro studies suggest that direct inhibition of *AKT1* or *PIK3CA* may be useful for Proteus syndrome (clinical trial in progress) and PROS.[28,83]

Understanding how mutations in these genes intersect with 1 signaling pathway explains the similarity among their clinical presentations and provides rationale for practical therapeutic approaches. Further, recognizing how mosaic involvement leads to variations in patterning explains the patchy and often asymmetric distribution of cutaneous and systemic involvement. The study of mosaic conditions along this pathway may also provide insights into the role of the PI3K/PTEN/AKT/TSC/mTORC1 pathway in skin biology, thereby improving understanding of common dermatologic problems.

REFERENCES

1. Biesecker LG, Spinner NB. A genomic view of mosaicism and human disease. Nat Rev Genet 2013;14: 307–20.
2. Happle R. Mosaicism in human skin understanding nevi, nevoid skin disorders, and cutaneous neoplasia. Dordrecht (Netherlands): Springer; 2013.
3. Happle R. The categories of cutaneous mosaicism: a proposed classification. Am J Med Genet A 2016;170:452–9.
4. Laplante M, Sabatini DM. mTOR signaling in growth control and disease. Cell 2012;149:274–93.
5. Dazert E, Hall MN. mTOR signaling in disease. Curr Opin Cell Biol 2011;23:744–55.
6. Inoki K, Li Y, Zhu T, et al. TSC2 is phosphorylated and inhibited by Akt and suppresses mTOR signalling. Nat Cell Biol 2002;4:648–57.
7. Huang J, Manning BD. A complex interplay between Akt, TSC2 and the two mTOR complexes. Biochem Soc Trans 2009;37:217–22.
8. Nguyen D, Turner JT, Olsen C, et al. Cutaneous manifestations of proteus syndrome: correlations with general clinical severity. Arch Dermatol 2004; 140:947–53.
9. Keppler-Noreuil KM, Sapp JC, Lindhurst MJ, et al. Clinical delineation and natural history of the PIK3CA-related overgrowth spectrum. Am J Med Genet A 2014;164:1713–33.
10. Mester J, Eng C. When overgrowth bumps into cancer: the PTEN-opathies. Am J Med Genet C Semin Med Genet 2013;163C(2):114–21.
11. Tyburczy ME, Dies KA, Glass J, et al. Mosaic and intronic mutations in TSC1/TSC2 explain the majority of TSC patients with no mutation identified by conventional testing. PLoS Genet 2015;11:e1005637.
12. Seibert D, Hong CH, Takeuchi F, et al. Recognition of tuberous sclerosis in adult women: delayed presentation with life-threatening consequences. Ann Intern Med 2011;154:806–13. W-294.
13. Cornu M, Albert V, Hall MN. mTOR in aging, metabolism, and cancer. Curr Opin Genet Dev 2013;23: 53–62.

14. Zhang H, Stallock JP, Ng JC, et al. Regulation of cellular growth by the Drosophila target of rapamycin dTOR. Genes Dev 2000;14:2712–24.

15. Rosner M, Hanneder M, Siegel N, et al. The mTOR pathway and its role in human genetic diseases. Mutat Res 2008;659:284–92.

16. Simpson L, Parsons R. PTEN: life as a tumor suppressor. Exp Cell Res 2001;264:29–41.

17. Maehama T, Dixon JE. The tumor suppressor, PTEN/MMAC1, dephosphorylates the lipid second messenger, phosphatidylinositol 3,4,5-trisphosphate. J Biol Chem 1998;273:13375–8.

18. Zhang Y, Gao X, Saucedo LJ, et al. Rheb is a direct target of the tuberous sclerosis tumour suppressor proteins. Nat Cell Biol 2003;5:578–81.

19. Pritchard CC, Smith C, Marushchak T, et al. A mosaic PTEN mutation causing Cowden syndrome identified by deep sequencing. Genet Med 2013;15:1004–7.

20. Salo-Mullen EE, Shia J, Brownell I, et al. Mosaic partial deletion of the PTEN gene in a patient with Cowden syndrome. Fam Cancer 2014;13(3):459–67.

21. Happle R. Type 2 segmental Cowden disease vs. proteus syndrome. Br J Dermatol 2007;156:1089–90.

22. Caux F, Plauchu H, Chibon F, et al. Segmental overgrowth, lipomatosis, arteriovenous malformation and epidermal nevus (SOLAMEN) syndrome is related to mosaic PTEN nullizygosity. Eur J Hum Genet 2007; 15:767–73.

23. Verhoef S, Bakker L, Tempelaars AM, et al. High rate of mosaicism in tuberous sclerosis complex. Am J Hum Genet 1999;64:1632–7.

24. Bader AG, Kang S, Vogt PK. Cancer-specific mutations in PIK3CA are oncogenic in vivo. Proc Natl Acad Sci U S A 2006;103:1475–9.

25. Sun M, Wang G, Paciga JE, et al. AKT1/PKBalpha kinase is frequently elevated in human cancers and its constitutive activation is required for oncogenic transformation in NIH3T3 cells. Am J Pathol 2001; 159:431–7.

26. Lindhurst MJ, Sapp JC, Teer JK, et al. A mosaic activating mutation in AKT1 associated with the Proteus syndrome. N Engl J Med 2011;365:611–9.

27. Kurek KC, Luks VL, Ayturk UM, et al. Somatic mosaic activating mutations in PIK3CA cause CLOVES syndrome. Am J Hum Genet 2012;90: 1108–15.

28. Lindhurst MJ, Yourick MR, Yu Y, et al. Repression of AKT signaling by ARQ 092 in cells and tissues from patients with Proteus syndrome. Sci Rep 2015;5: 17162.

29. Orloff MS, He X, Peterson C, et al. Germline PIK3CA and AKT1 mutations in Cowden and Cowden-like syndromes. Am J Hum Genet 2013;92:76–80.

30. Keppler-Noreuil KM, Rios JJ, Parker VE, et al. PIK3CA-related overgrowth spectrum (PROS): diagnostic and testing eligibility criteria, differential diagnosis, and evaluation. Am J Med Genet A 2015;167A:287–95.

31. Sapp JC, Turner JT, van de Kamp JM, et al. Newly delineated syndrome of congenital lipomatous overgrowth, vascular malformations, and epidermal nevi (CLOVE syndrome) in seven patients. Am J Med Genet A 2007;143A:2944–58.

32. Twede JV, Turner JT, Biesecker LG, et al. Evolution of skin lesions in Proteus syndrome. J Am Acad Dermatol 2005;52:834–8.

33. Carty MJ, Taghinia A, Upton J. Overgrowth conditions: a diagnostic and therapeutic conundrum. Hand Clin 2009;25:229–45.

34. Chakrabarti N, Chattopadhyay C, Bhuban M, et al. Proteus syndrome: a rare cause of gigantic limb. Indian Dermatol Online J 2014;5:193–5.

35. Happle R. The group of epidermal nevus syndromes part II. Less well defined phenotypes. J Am Acad Dermatol 2010;63:25–30 [quiz: 1–2].

36. Happle R. Mosaicism in human skin. Understanding the patterns and mechanisms. Arch Dermatol 1993; 129:1460–70.

37. Biesecker L. The challenges of Proteus syndrome: diagnosis and management. Eur J Hum Genet 2006;14:1151–7.

38. Hafner C, Lopez-Knowles E, Luis NM, et al. Oncogenic PIK3CA mutations occur in epidermal nevi and seborrheic keratoses with a characteristic mutation pattern. Proc Natl Acad Sci U S A 2007;104: 13450–4.

39. Groesser L, Herschberger E, Landthaler M, et al. FGFR3, PIK3CA and RAS mutations in benign lichenoid keratosis. Br J Dermatol 2012;166:784–8.

40. Luks VL, Kamitaki N, Vivero MP, et al. Lymphatic and other vascular malformative/overgrowth disorders are caused by somatic mutations in PIK3CA. J Pediatr 2015;166:1048–54.e1–5.

41. Castillo SD, Tzouanacou E, Zaw-Thin M, et al. Somatic activating mutations in Pik3ca cause sporadic venous malformations in mice and humans. Sci Transl Med 2016;8:332ra43.

42. Vahidnezhad H, Youssefian L, Uitto J. Klippel-Trenaunay syndrome belongs to the PIK3CA-related overgrowth spectrum (PROS). Exp Dermatol 2016; 25:17–9.

43. Eng C. PTEN hamartoma tumor syndrome (PHTS). In: Pagon RA, Adam MP, Ardinger HH, et al, editors. Seattle (WA): GeneReviews(R); © 1993–2016 University of Washington, (http://www.genereviews. org/) Initial Posting: November 29, 2001; Last Update: June 2, 2016.

44. Pilarski R, Burt R, Kohlman W, et al. Cowden syndrome and the PTEN hamartoma tumor syndrome: systematic review and revised diagnostic criteria. J Natl Cancer Inst 2013;105:1607–16.

45. Marsh DJ, Coulon V, Lunetta KL, et al. Mutation spectrum and genotype-phenotype analyses in

Cowden disease and Bannayan-Zonana syndrome, two hamartoma syndromes with germline PTEN mutation. Hum Mol Genet 1998;7:507–15.

46. Marsh DJ, Kum JB, Lunetta KL, et al. PTEN mutation spectrum and genotype-phenotype correlations in Bannayan-Riley-Ruvalcaba syndrome suggest a single entity with Cowden syndrome. Hum Mol Genet 1999;8:1461–72.

47. Molho-Pessach V, Schaffer JV. Blaschko lines and other patterns of cutaneous mosaicism. Clin Dermatol 2011;29:205–25.

48. Happle R. A rule concerning the segmental manifestation of autosomal dominant skin disorders. Review of clinical examples providing evidence for dichotomous types of severity. Arch Dermatol 1997;133:1505–9.

49. Kouzak SS, Mendes MS, Costa IM. Cutaneous mosaicisms: concepts, patterns and classifications. An Bras Dermatol 2013;88:507–17.

50. Gammon A, Jasperson K, Pilarski R, et al. PTEN mosaicism with features of Cowden syndrome. Clin Genet 2013;84:593–5.

51. Happle R. Linear Cowden nevus: a new distinct epidermal nevus. Eur J Dermatol 2007;17:133–6.

52. Kurek KC, Howard E, Tennant LB, et al. PTEN hamartoma of soft tissue: a distinctive lesion in PTEN syndromes. Am J Surg Pathol 2012;36:671–87.

53. Curatolo P, Bombardieri R, Jozwiak S. Tuberous sclerosis. Lancet 2008;372:657–68.

54. Napolioni V, Curatolo P. Genetics and molecular biology of tuberous sclerosis complex. Curr Genomics 2008;9:475–87.

55. Northrup H, Krueger DA, International Tuberous Sclerosis Complex Consensus Group. Tuberous sclerosis complex diagnostic criteria update: recommendations of the 2012 Iinternational Tuberous Sclerosis Complex Consensus Conference. Pediatr Neurol 2013;49:243–54.

56. Nathan N, Tyburczy ME, Hamieh L, et al. Nipple angiofibromas with loss of TSC2 are associated with tuberous sclerosis complex. J Invest Dermatol 2016; 136:535–8.

57. Teng JM, Cowen EW, Wataya-Kaneda M, et al. Dermatologic and dental aspects of the 2012 International Tuberous Sclerosis Complex Consensus Statements. JAMA Dermatol 2014;150:1095–101.

58. Sparling JD, Hong CH, Brahim JS, et al. Oral findings in 58 adults with tuberous sclerosis complex. J Am Acad Dermatol 2007;56:786–90.

59. Dabora SL, Jozwiak S, Franz DN, et al. Mutational analysis in a cohort of 224 tuberous sclerosis patients indicates increased severity of TSC2, compared with TSC1, disease in multiple organs. Am J Hum Genet 2001;68:64–80.

60. Kozlowski P, Roberts P, Dabora S, et al. Identification of 54 large deletions/duplications in TSC1 and TSC2 using MLPA, and genotype-phenotype correlations. Hum Genet 2007;121:389–400.

61. Au KS, Williams AT, Roach ES, et al. Genotype/phenotype correlation in 325 individuals referred for a diagnosis of tuberous sclerosis complex in the United States. Genet Med 2007;9:88–100.

62. Delaney SP, Julian LM, Stanford WL. The neural crest lineage as a driver of disease heterogeneity in tuberous sclerosis complex and lymphangioleiomyomatosis. Front Cell Dev Biol 2014;2:69.

63. Hall MR, Kovach BT, Miller JL. Unilateral facial angiofibromas without other evidence of tuberous sclerosis: case report and review of the literature. Cutis 2007;80:284–8.

64. Boronat S, Caruso P, Thiele EA. Absence of subependymal nodules in patients with tubers suggests possible neuroectodermal mosaicism in tuberous sclerosis complex. Dev Med Child Neurol 2014; 56(12):1207–11.

65. Boronat S, Shaaya E, Doherty C, et al. Tuberous sclerosis complex without tubers and subependymal nodules: a phenotype-genotype study. Clin Genet 2014;86(2):149–54.

66. Wee JS, Mortimer PS, Lindhurst MJ, et al. A limited form of proteus syndrome with bilateral plantar cerebriform collagenomas and varicose veins secondary to a mosaic AKT1 mutation. JAMA Dermatol 2014; 150(9):990–3.

67. Lindhurst MJ, Wang JA, Bloomhardt HM, et al. AKT1 gene mutation levels are correlated with the type of dermatologic lesions in patients with Proteus syndrome. J Invest Dermatol 2014;134:543–6.

68. Li S, Takeuchi F, Wang JA, et al. Mesenchymal-epithelial interactions involving epiregulin in tuberous sclerosis complex hamartomas. Proc Natl Acad Sci U S A 2008;105:3539–44.

69. Tyburczy ME, Wang JA, Li S, et al. Sun exposure causes somatic second-hit mutations and angiofibroma development in tuberous sclerosis complex. Hum Mol Genet 2014;23:2023–9.

70. Wieland I, Tinschert S, Zenker M. High-level somatic mosaicism of AKT1 c.49G>A mutation in skin scrapings from epidermal nevi enables non-invasive molecular diagnosis in patients with Proteus syndrome. Am J Med Genet A 2013;161A:889–91.

71. Sancak O, Nellist M, Goedbloed M, et al. Mutational analysis of the TSC1 and TSC2 genes in a diagnostic setting: genotype–phenotype correlations and comparison of diagnostic DNA techniques in tuberous sclerosis complex. Eur J Hum Genet 2005; 13:731–41.

72. Rasmussen M, Sunde L, Weigert KP, et al. Segmental overgrowth syndrome due to an activating PIK3CA mutation identified in affected muscle tissue by exome sequencing. Am J Med Genet A 2014;164A: 1318–21.

73. Nathan N, Burke K, Trickett C, et al. The adult phenotype of tuberous sclerosis complex in men. Acta Derm Venereol 2016;96(2):278–80.

74. Krueger DA, Northrup H, International Tuberous Sclerosis Complex Consensus Group. Tuberous sclerosis complex surveillance and management: recommendations of the 2012 International Tuberous Sclerosis Complex Consensus Conference. Pediatr Neurol 2013;49:255–65.

75. Bjornsson J, Short MP, Kwiatkowski DJ, et al. Tuberous sclerosis-associated renal cell carcinoma. Clinical, pathological, and genetic features. Am J Pathol 1996;149:1201–8.

76. Lapunzina P. Risk of tumorigenesis in overgrowth syndromes: a comprehensive review. Am J Med Genet C Semin Med Genet 2005;137C:53–71.

77. Hoyme HE, Seaver LH, Jones KL, et al. Isolated hemihyperplasia (hemihypertrophy): report of a prospective multicenter study of the incidence of neoplasia and review. Am J Med Genet 1998;79: 274–8.

78. Clericuzio CL, Martin RA. Diagnostic criteria and tumor screening for individuals with isolated hemihyperplasia. Genet Med 2009;11:220–2.

79. Castiglioni C, Bertini E, Orellana P, et al. Activating PIK3CA somatic mutation in congenital unilateral isolated muscle overgrowth of the upper extremity. Am J Med Genet A 2014;164A:2365–9.

80. Nathan N, Wang JA, Li S, et al. Improvement of tuberous sclerosis complex (TSC) skin tumors during long-term treatment with oral sirolimus. J Am Acad Dermatol 2015;73:802–8.

81. Schmid GL, Kassner F, Uhlig HH, et al. Sirolimus treatment of severe PTEN hamartoma tumor syndrome: case report and in vitro studies. Pediatr Res 2014;75:527–34.

82. Fogel AL, Hill S, Teng JM. Advances in the therapeutic use of mammalian target of rapamycin (mTOR) inhibitors in dermatology. J Am Acad Dermatol 2015;72:879–89.

83. Loconte DC, Grossi V, Bozzao C, et al. Molecular and functional characterization of three different postzygotic mutations in PIK3CA-related overgrowth spectrum (PROS) patients: effects on PI3K/AKT/mTOR signaling and sensitivity to PIK3 inhibitors. PLoS One 2015;10:e0123092.

Understanding Inherited Cylindromas
Clinical Implications of Gene Discovery

Anna Dubois, BSc, MBChB[a], Kirsty Hodgson, BSc, MRes[b],
Neil Rajan, MBBS, PhD[b,c],*

KEYWORDS

- CYLD • Cylindroma • Spiradenoma • *CYLD* cutaneous syndrome • Brooke-Spiegler syndrome

KEY POINTS

- Cylindromas, trichoepitheliomas, and spiradenomas are tumors of the skin appendages occurring in familial cylindromatosis, multiple familial trichoepithelioma, and Brooke-Spiegler syndrome.
- The tumor-suppressor gene *CYLD* was discovered in 2000 and mutations in this gene are responsible for the development of the three tumor syndromes, collectively termed CYLD cutaneous syndrome.
- This dominantly inherited syndrome is highly penetrant; however, severity may vary.
- Molecular characterization of CYLD function in skin biology has led to new mechanistic insights into tumorigenesis in the care of these patients and paved the way for novel therapeutic strategies.

INTRODUCTION

Tumors of the skin appendages occur sporadically and as part of inherited syndromes. Although these tumors have been described in the medical literature for many years, it is only recently that advances in genetics have allowed clinicians to further understand the origin of these lesions and delineate the clinical syndromes with which they are associated.

Skin appendages are derived from the embryonic ectoderm[1] and include three histologically distinct structures: (1) the pilosebaceous unit (hair follicle and sebaceous glands), (2) the eccrine sweat gland, and (3) the apocrine gland. Tumors of these adnexal structures are classified according to their differentiation as follicular, sebaceous, eccrine or apocrine. Cylindromas are a type of skin appendage tumor thought to arise from hair follicle stem cells.[2] Most present as papules on the skin, mainly on the face and scalp, which can be difficult to differentiate clinically. Diagnosis is often made on histologic assessment of skin biopsy. Although found only rarely on a sporadic basis, cylindromas are the characteristic tumor occurring in multiple numbers in several syndromes.

The autosomal-dominant condition familial cylindromatosis (FC; OMIM 132700) is now known to be caused by a germline mutation in the gene *CYLD*. The first reported case of a patient with FC was described by Ancell in 1842[3] (**Fig. 1**) and since then cylindroma, a benign skin appendage tumor, has continued to fascinate, with new mechanistic understandings and insights unfolding up to the present day.

Disclosure Statement: The authors have nothing to disclose.
[a] Department of Dermatology, Royal Victoria Infirmary, Queen Victoria Road, Newcastle upon Tyne NE1 4LP, UK; [b] Institute of Genetic Medicine, Newcastle University, International Centre for Life, Central Parkway, Newcastle upon Tyne, NE1 3BZ, UK; [c] Department of Dermatology, Royal Victoria Infirmary, Queen Victoria Road, Newcastle upon Tyne NE1 4LP, UK
* Corresponding author. Institute of Genetic Medicine, Newcastle University, Newcastle upon Tyne, NE1 3BZ, United Kingdom.
E-mail address: neil.rajan@ncl.ac.uk

Dermatol Clin 35 (2017) 61–71
http://dx.doi.org/10.1016/j.det.2016.08.002
0733-8635/17/© 2016 Elsevier Inc. All rights reserved.

In addition to FC, cylindromas are also found in two additional related tumor syndromes. Multiple familial trichoepitheliomas (MFT; OMIM 601606) is a condition defined by the trichoepithelioma, a small skin-colored tumor mainly found on the face, with cylindromas coexisting in lower numbers. Brooke-Spiegler syndrome (BSS; OMIM 605041) is considered an overlap between FC and MFT, and here cylindroma and trichoepithelioma occur together with another related tumor, spiradenoma. Key early descriptions of these conditions, which led to the eponymous "BSS," include a report of a British family with multiple trichoepitheliomas by Brooke in 1892,[4] and an Austrian case of cylindromas by Spiegler in 1899.[5]

Cue forward to the year 2000, and the *CYLD* gene was discovered by positional cloning and Sanger sequencing. In-depth study of pedigrees with FC using a genetic technique called "linkage analysis" pinpointed the *CYLD* locus to chromosome 16q, which led subsequently to identification of the gene itself. With this came the confirmation that FC, MFT, and BSS are not in fact separate entities, but overlapping phenotypes resulting from mutations leading to loss of functional CYLD. *CYLD* functions as a recessive tumor-suppressor gene, and cylindromas show loss of heterozygosity at the *CYLD* locus as a result of a somatic second-hit on top of a pre-existing germline mutation.[6] Collectively, these conditions may be termed CYLD cutaneous syndrome, because individual labels do not prognosticate.[7]

The discovery of *CYLD* paved the way for several major steps forward that have occurred in the past 16 years. The mechanisms of tumor formation in the skin can now be investigated and understood on a molecular genetic basis. In addition, the wider role of *CYLD* has been explored and the cell signaling pathways it regulates have become better understood.

This article provides an overview of the features of the cutaneous tumors that arise in *CYLD* mutation carriers. Current knowledge of the gene and its function are reviewed, before considering how insights gained from this scientific information may be used toward investigating novel therapeutic strategies in patients.

SKIN TUMORS ASSOCIATED WITH GERMLINE CYLINDROMATOSIS MUTATIONS
Clinical Features

Cylindromas are benign, well-circumscribed, smooth, pale pink nodular tumors, often with arborizing vessels visible (Fig. 2). The tumors are slow growing and vary in size from a few millimeters to more than 5 cm. In severe cases, tumors may cover most of the scalp, which led to the previously used term "turban tumor."[8] Spiradenomas are benign nodular tumors that are often blue-black in color. They tend to be painful and can

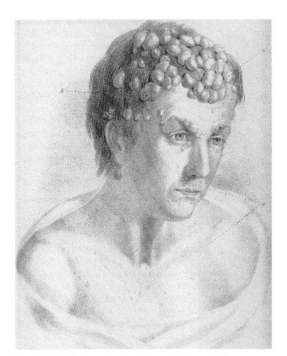

Fig. 1. The first patient with multiple cylindromas reported in the medical literature, a 52-year-old English woman, described by Ancell in 1842. She presented with metastatic disease and had a strong family history of cutaneous tumors. (*From* Ancell H. History of a remarkable case of tumors, developed on the head and face; accompanied with a similar disease in the abdomen. Med Chir Trans 1842;25:227; with permission.)

grow up to 10 cm in diameter. Trichoepitheliomas are benign tumors, presenting as skin-colored papules. They are mainly found on the face, and are small, usually no more than 2 to 5 mm across. All benign, these skin appendage tumors occur in FC, MFT, and BSS.

Tumors usually start to occur in the second or third decades and accumulate throughout adulthood[9] and most patients with a *CYLD* mutation present with more than one tumor type. Mutations in *CYLD* are transmitted in an autosomal-dominant fashion and affect males and females equally. The expression and penetrance of tumor development can vary, however, and there have been reports of a female preponderance to tumors in mutation carriers.[10]

Histologic Features

Cylindromas are thought to arise from precursor cells in the hair follicle epithelium,[2,11] although previously there has been debate as to the cell of origin, and whether they derive from the follicular, apocrine, or eccrine line (see **Fig. 2**).[12] Cylindromas are nonencapsulated nodular tumors extending into the dermis. They consist of well-defined nests of basaloid cells in a jigsaw pattern, separated by an eosinophilic basement membrane. The term cylindroma is based on the description of the nests of basaloid cells that resemble cylinders when cut in cross-section.[13] Spiradenomas lack the organized structure of cylindromas. They comprise a dense basophilic cellular pattern, vessels may be obvious, and there is often a lymphocytic infiltrate. Some individual lesions show histologic features consistent with both cylindroma and spiradenoma, and have been given the overlap term spiradenocylindromas.[14,15] Indeed, cylindroma and spiradenoma may represent extremes of a spectrum of the same tumor type, with the transition to spiradenoma being influenced by epigenetic modulation of cell-signaling pathways, such as Wnt.[16] Both tumor patterns express cytokeratins seen in hair follicles, such as CK14[17] and CK17, and also have regions where cytokeratins seen in eccrine glands are present, such as CK18 and CK77 (**Fig. 3**). Trichoepitheliomas are nontender skin-colored nodules, with islands of basaloid cells, sometimes displaying peripheral palisading.

Tumor-Associated Morbidity

Although benign, presence of these tumors carries significant morbidity for *CYLD* mutation carriers. They can frequently be painful, or may bleed or ulcerate, necessitating removal by repeated episodes of surgery. The tumors and the surgical procedures to reduce tumor burden can be disfiguring. Tumors occurring in the ear canal, a favored site for tumor formation, can occlude patency of the canal, resulting in a conductive deafness. Patients can develop painful spiradenomas within pubic skin, resulting in sexual dysfunction. When the tumors cover the head extensively, the scalp skin may need to be grafted and reconstructed.[18] In addition to the physical burden of disease, psychological consequences including depression may occur in those affected.

Malignant Transformation of Benign Tumors

Cylindroma and spiradenoma may undergo malignant transformation into cylindrocarcinoma and spiradenocarcinoma, respectively. This happens infrequently, with fewer than 50 reported cases in the literature.[19] Malignant change is more likely to arise in cylindromas occurring as a result of a *CYLD* mutation than in solitary sporadic tumors[19] because there are many more lesions in these patients. Clinical features that raise suspicion of malignant transformation include ulceration, rapid growth, pain, bleeding, color change, and the lesion becoming tethered or fixed.[20] This may

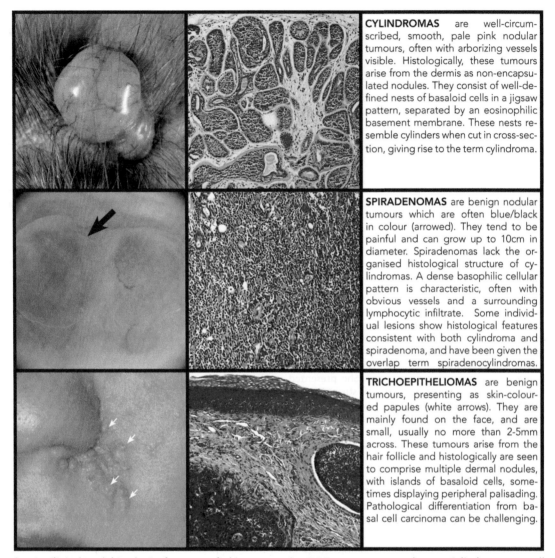

CYLINDROMAS are well-circumscribed, smooth, pale pink nodular tumours, often with arborizing vessels visible. Histologically, these tumours arise from the dermis as non-encapsulated nodules. They consist of well-defined nests of basaloid cells in a jigsaw pattern, separated by an eosinophilic basement membrane. These nests resemble cylinders when cut in cross-section, giving rise to the term cylindroma.

SPIRADENOMAS are benign nodular tumours which are often blue/black in colour (arrowed). They tend to be painful and can grow up to 10cm in diameter. Spiradenomas lack the organised histological structure of cylindromas. A dense basophilic cellular pattern is characteristic, often with obvious vessels and a surrounding lymphocytic infiltrate. Some individual lesions show histological features consistent with both cylindroma and spiradenoma, and have been given the overlap term spiradenocylindromas.

TRICHOEPITHELIOMAS are benign tumours, presenting as skin-coloured papules (white arrows). They are mainly found on the face, and are small, usually no more than 2-5mm across. These tumours arise from the hair follicle and histologically are seen to comprise multiple dermal nodules, with islands of basaloid cells, sometimes displaying peripheral palisading. Pathological differentiation from basal cell carcinoma can be challenging.

Fig. 2. Clinical and histologic features of skin tumors in CYLD cutaneous syndrome. Cylindroma: a well-circumscribed, nodular lesion with visible arborizing vessels arising from the scalp. Stain shows typical nests of basaloid cells arranged in a cylinder pattern (hematoxylin-eosin, original magnification ×10). Spiradenoma: a nodular lesion with a characteristic blue hue (*black arrow*). Stain shows a disorganized structure, with densely packed basophilc cells (hematoxylin-eosin, original magnification ×10). Trichoepithelioma: Small skin-colored papules occurring in the typical melolabial distribution (*white arrows*). Stain shows a nodular arrangement of basaloid cells in the dermis (hematoxylin-eosin, original magnification ×10).

inform clinical advice given to patients on when to report changing lesions to their dermatologist. Tumors invade locally and may also metastasize to organs including the stomach, thyroid, liver, and lung. Histologically, cylindrocarcinoma may display highly pleomorphic irregular cells with atypical mitoses and disruption of the usual 'jigsaw' pattern.[21] Spiradenocarcinomas are composed of solid islands of tumor cells that may show either a squamous or a basaloid pattern.[22] Basal cell carcinomas have been reported to occur in conjunction with trichoepitheliomas,[23] but the direct association between these tumors is unusual. Trichoblastoma, a variant of trichoepithelioma, has been reported to transform into trichoblastic carcinoma,[24] which can metastasize.

Mosaic Presentations

In some patients, the tumors associated with a mutation in the CYLD gene are found in a distinctive linear arrangement,[25,26] corresponding to the lines of Blaschko.[27] These are areas of skin that each arise from a single epidermal cell.[28] If a somatic

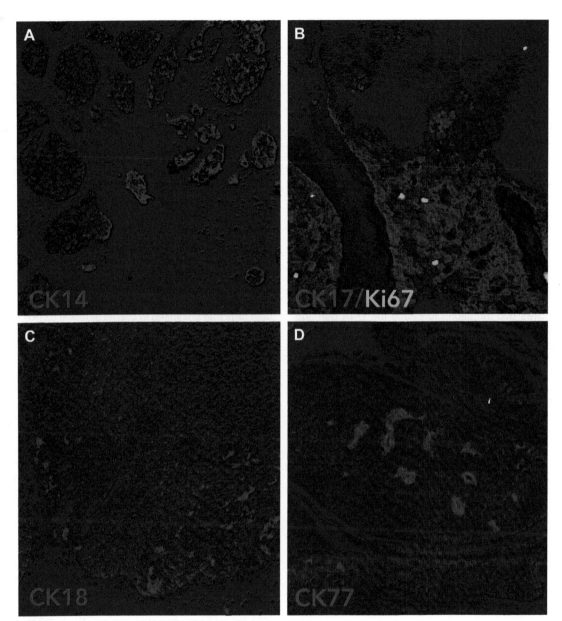

Fig. 3. Expression of hair follicle and eccrine duct keratins in cylindroma frozen tissue sections. (*A*) Cytokeratin 14 (CK14) is widely expressed in tumor cells. (*B*) Cytokeratin 17 (CK17) is also widely expressed in tumors (*red stain*). Few cells express ki67 (*green stain*) indicating low proliferation. (*C*) Small areas within cylindromas express cytokeratin 18 (CK18). (*D*) Areas of ductal differentiation within tumors express cytokeratin 77 (CK77). DAPI (4′,6-dia-midine-2′-phenylindole dihydrochloride) was used for nuclear staining.

mutation in *CYLD* occurs at the postzygotic stage of embryonic development in an individual with a background of a pre-existing germline mutation, then all the cells arising from the single mutated cell are homozygous for a mutation in *CYLD* and have the propensity to develop cutaneous tumors.[29]

Associated Tumors

A small proportion of patients, estimated at less than 5%, develop low-grade salivary gland tumors, typically membranous basal cell adenoma.[30]

CYLINDROMATOSIS AS A CAUSATIVE GENE FOR SKIN APPENDAGE TUMORS
Discovery of Cylindromatosis

Accurate pedigrees of families with syndromes causing cylindromas and related tumors showed early on that these were Mendelian, inherited in an autosomal-dominant fashion. The knowledge that these syndromes were associated with a single gene, rather than being complex disorders resulting from both multiple genetic and environmental influences, meant that discovery of the causative gene was possible. The technique for gene discovery at the time used linkage studies, based on matching the inheritance pattern of a condition in a family with specific genetic markers, which are also inherited and can be tracked. The CYLD gene locus was first mapped to chromosome 16q12 to 13 in 1996[31] using this technique, and the CYLD gene was subsequently discovered to be causative for BSS and FC in 2000[32,33] and for MFT in 2004,[34] using Sanger sequencing.

CYLD is a tumor-suppressor gene. Although a mutation in CYLD is inherited in an autosomal-dominant manner, at the molecular level, the gene is known as a recessive oncogene. Following the principle of the two-hit hypothesis,[6] a cell requires two mutations to cause the DNA damage leading to tumor development. When a germline mutation (from conception) is present, an individual has cells that are heterozygous for that mutation, that is, one copy of the gene in question is already damaged. If a second mutation occurs to the additional copy of the gene, which may happen as a random event resulting from DNA damage that occurs as part of normal life, this can lead to the cell becoming neoplastic. The tumor then displays loss of heterozygosity for the gene in question, as was found in CYLD as part of the discovery process. These steps forward in understanding were a major turning point in clinicians' perceptions of these disorders.

In addition to mutations in CYLD, sporadic cylindromas have been found to carry the MYB-NFIB gene fusion, which also plays an important role in the development of adenoid cystic carcinoma, a rare malignancy primarily found in the salivary gland.[35]

Cylindromatosis Function

The CYLD gene (GenBank number NM_015247) spans 56kb and is composed of 20 exons and 19 introns.[36] The gene encodes the protein CYLD, 956 amino acids in length with a molecular weight of 107 kDa. It contains three cytoskeletal-associated protein-glycine-conserved domains, and one ubiquitin carboxyl-terminal hydrolase domain. It also has two proline-rich segments constituting an SH3 domain and four finger-like metal binding domains. CYLD is expressed predominantly in the fetal brain, testis, and skeletal muscle and is also found at lower levels in many adult tissues including the liver, heart, kidney,

spleen, ovary, and lung. In the skin CYLD is expressed in hair follicles, epidermis, and eccrine glands.[2,37] Despite this widespread expression, tumors associated with CYLD occur primarily in the skin, suggesting that additional factors other than the expression pattern are important in tumor development.

Since CYLD was discovered, interesting insights have been gained into the CYLD protein, in particular its function in controlling inflammation and cell proliferation. CYLD is classified as belonging to a family of enzymes called deubiquitinases, which have five classes. The cysteine protease class, of which CYLD is a member, is further divided based on protease domains, and CYLD is in the ubiquitin-specific protease subclass. Proteases in this family contribute to posttranslational modification of proteins. CYLD catalyzes the removal of a protein tag called ubiquitin from different substrates. CYLD is a deubiquitinase with specificity for ubiquitin tags that are linked in chains at lysine 63 (K63-linked polyubiquitin chains). This is important in regulating cell-signaling pathways and protein stability via processes including DNA repair, endocytosis, and proteosomal degradation.[38]

In continuing to explore the functions of CYLD, investigating its interaction with nuclear factor (NF)-κB signaling has proved to be an area of importance. NF-κB is a family of five transcription factors that regulate genes involved in a wide range of functions, including facilitating the response of cells to signals that prevent apoptosis, regulation of inflammation and cell proliferation,[39] and contributing to the process of tumor suppression.[40] NF-κB also has a role in the molecular control of hair follicle development and maintenance.[41]

CYLD has been shown to negatively regulate the tumor necrosis factor-α– associated canonical NF-κB signaling pathway (Fig. 4). Some of the specific substrates that CYLD acts on within this pathway have been identified. CYLD removes K63-linked polyubiquitin chains from TRAF2, TRAF6, and the regulatory subunit of the IKK complex, NEMO.[42,43] Removal of K63-linked ubiquitin from these substrates prevents activation of the IKK complex. When activated, the IKK complex phosphorylates IκBα, an inhibitory protein that sequesters the NF-κB transcription factors RELA/p65 and NF-κB1/p50 in the cytoplasm. Phosphorylation of IκBα results in its degradation by the proteasome, freeing p65 and p50 to enter the nucleus to regulate gene expression. In addition, CYLD also deubiquitinates other components of the NF-κB pathway including MAP3K7[44] and BCL3, affecting cellular proliferation via BCL3 nuclear translocation and cyclin D1 upregulation.[45] Removal of polyubiquitin chains from these

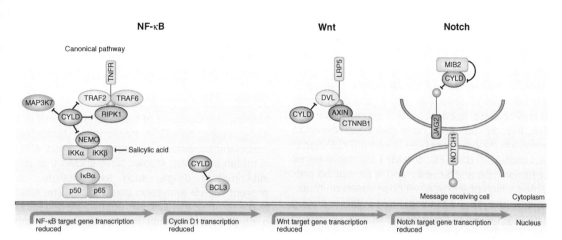

Fig. 4. A schematic representation showing some of the pathways negatively regulated by CYLD. In the canonical NF-κB signaling pathway, CYLD removes lysine 63 linked ubiquitin molecules from TRAF2, TRAF6, and NEMO to prevent downstream activation of the IKK complex. When the IKK complex is inactive, the NF-κB transcription factors p65 and p50 are inhibited by IκBα within the cytoplasm. CYLD also deubiquitinates BCL3, preventing BCL3 from translocating to the nucleus where it acts as a transcriptional coactivator with p50 or p52 to increase expression of genes, such as cyclin D1. In the Wnt signaling pathway, CYLD deubiquitinates Disheveled (DVL), which prevents downstream activation of the transcriptional coactivator β-catenin (CTNNB1). Notch signaling via JAG2 is attenuated because of the interaction of CYLD with MIB2.

substrates attenuates NF-κB signaling, leading ultimately to apoptosis.[46] CYLD is known, in addition, to negatively regulate the c-Jun N-terminal kinase signaling pathway, also involved in cell survival. The role of CYLD in this pathway is thought to be connected to TRAF2 ubiquitination.[47] Negative regulation by CYLD of other pathways important in cell signaling including Wnt,[48] Notch,[49] and TGFB1[50] also plays a role in development of inflammation and cancer.

Mutations in cylindromatosis

Over 100 mutations in *CYLD* have been reported.[51] Many of these originate from the United Kingdom or United States, but a diverse range of geographic locations are also represented. Frameshift and nonsense mutations predominate, but splice site and missense mutations have also been reported, and two in-frame deletions.[52] The mutations typically are predicted to cause truncation of the *CYLD* protein product. Mutations in *CYLD* have been found to mainly occur in the 3′ two-thirds of the coding sequence between exons 9 to 20 (**Fig. 5**). Although the number of reported *CYLD* mutations is regularly being added to in the literature, there is still a lack of understanding with regard to the effect any particular mutation has on the phenotype.[53] There does not seem to be significant correlation between where the mutation is found on the gene or the type of mutation, and the tumor type

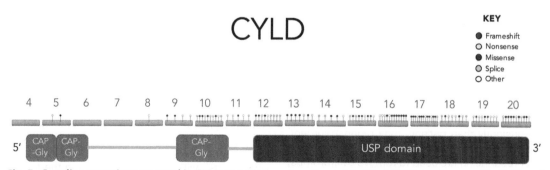

Fig. 5. Germline mutations reported in *CYLD* mutation carriers. Exons 4 to 20 of *CYLD* are shown, with "lollipop" markers denoting reported mutations. *Red circles* indicate frameshift mutations, *yellow circles* indicate nonsense mutations, *purple circles* indicate missense mutations, *blue circles* indicate splice site mutations, and *white circles* indicate other/unknown types of mutations. The *gray boxes* indicate the positions of the three cytoskeleton-associated protein glycine-rich (CAP-Gly) domains of CYLD. The *purple box* indicates the position of the CYLD catalytic ubiquitin specific protease (USP) protein domain.

that presents.[54] Neither is it possible to predict severity of disease in different carriers of the same mutation as seen in variation in multigenerational pedigrees. Carriers of the same mutation often have clinical manifestations that vary significantly in their severity of tumor burden present.[55] It is possible that modifier genes, and differences in environment, account for this phenotypic variation. Intronic mutations have also been shown to contribute to the phenotype in some CYLD mutation carriers.[56] BSS, FC, and MFT overlap in terms of tumor type and severity and it cannot be predicted which phenotype will arise based on mutational analysis, meaning that differentiating clinically between these conditions is of limited use. CYLD cutaneous syndrome is hence proposed as a collective term for these conditions.[7]

Cylindromatosis in Other Tumors

Investigating the role of CYLD has increased understanding of other tumors. In addition to its role in skin appendage tumors, CYLD acts as a tumor suppressor in several other cancers, in which somatic mutations may affect NF-κB signaling. Reduced expression of CYLD, thought to contribute to tumor pathogenesis, has been shown in cancers including melanoma,[57] bowel cancer,[58] lung cancer,[59] multiple myeloma,[60] hepatocellular carcinoma,[58] and prostate cancer[61] and are reviewed separately.[51]

MANAGEMENT OF TUMORS

With increasing knowledge of the pathogenesis of cutaneous tumors resulting from a mutation in the CYLD gene comes advances in their treatment. Although surgical management is still the most effective modality, steps forward in terms of medical therapeutic developments are on the horizon.

Surgical Management

The mainstay of tumor management in those with a CYLD mutation is surgical removal. Because patients may develop several tumors over a lifetime, repeated surgical procedures may be required. Because the tumors are benign, they do not have to be excised once the diagnosis is confirmed histologically, but if they are causing discomfort or are unsightly then patients may request surgery. Primary excision, curettage, electrosurgery, and laser resurfacing are used to remove cylindromas, spiradenomas, and trichoepitheliomas.[62]

Radiotherapy

Radiotherapy has previously been used to treat these tumors, but conventional wisdom in tumor biology dictates that use of radiotherapy may result in further DNA damage to cells already affected with a CYLD mutation and is therefore contraindicated. It may also increase the risk of further tumors developing in the surrounding skin.

Medical Management

Medical management of these tumors is still in its early stages. NF-κB, a transcription factor with antiapoptotic activity, is activated when CYLD is mutated. In vitro studies have shown that anti-inflammatory drugs, such as salicylate, can prevent NK-κB activation (see **Fig. 4**). The effectiveness of topical salicylic acid was evaluated in a study,[63] but overall the results were disappointing, with only 2 of 12 cylindromas showing complete remission. A case report[64] that trailed oral aspirin and adalimumab to block tumor necrosis factor activation of NF-κB showed a gradual improvement in lesions, but the patient was being treated concurrently with laser resurfacing. A future research direction may be to investigate the role of neurotrophic tyrosine receptor kinase signaling, which is a family implicated in tumorigenesis. Currently clinical trials are underway to establish the use of targeting TRK in cylindromas.

Malignant Tumors

Principles of management for tumors that have undergone malignant transformation are similar to those for other cutaneous malignances. Excision with an appropriate skin margin should be performed and imaging considered following discussion by a multidisciplinary team typically involving dermatologists, pathologists, oncologists, and radiologists.

Genetic Counseling

Genetic counseling is the process by which those with or at risk of inheriting a mutation in CYLD are advised of the nature of the condition, the risk of transmission and inheritance, and options for genetic testing and management of their risk. Genetic testing for CYLD mutations is performed in several scenarios, including in a patient with multiple cylindromas, spiradenomas, or trichoepitheliomas; an individual with a single cylindroma, spiradenoma, or trichoepithelioma in combination with an affected first-degree relative with any of these tumors; or an asymptomatic family member at 50% risk with a known mutation in the family. The counseling process is tailored to the particular situation of the patient.

When a pathogenic mutation in CYLD is identified in a patient who meets the criteria for testing, they have the advantage of knowing their diagnosis is confirmed, and can use the information for their benefit. Testing may also be requested by those at genetic risk to inform reproductive decisions, even if they do not have clinical signs of the condition. The oldest patient to develop a first tumor in the literature was 42 years of age.[65] In an unaffected patient within a family where a *CYLD* mutation is present, a negative result is useful because it rules out further transmission of the familial mutation and may inform family planning. A positive result in an unaffected individual, however, is more challenging to interpret. Because there is poor genotype-phenotype correlation, a positive result does not predict severity. Further work is needed to determine other influencing factors.

FUTURE DIRECTIONS

The discovery of *CYLD* as the causative gene in CYLD cutaneous syndrome marked the advent of genetic diagnosis and counseling. The progressive understanding of CYLD function, and the cell signaling pathways that CYLD regulates, has paved the way for the potential development of novel therapeutic approaches.

The apparent lack of genotype-phenotype correlation in *CYLD* mutation carriers suggests that modifier genes may be likely to play a role in contributing to the clinical phenotype. Discovery of these genes and information about their function in relation to *CYLD* may improve the accuracy of prognostic information that could be given to those with a *CYLD* mutation.

It is hoped that continual molecular dissection of this rare disease will provide benefits for patients with CYLD cutaneous syndrome and other patients with sporadic cancers where the tumor suppressor CYLD is mutated or repressed.

ACKNOWLEDGMENTS

N. Rajan is a Wellcome Intermediate Fellow. The authors thank Lutz Langbein for his gift of the CK77 antibody.

REFERENCES

1. Biggs LC, Mikkola ML. Early inductive events in ectodermal appendage morphogenesis. Semin Cell Dev Biol 2014;25-26:11–21.
2. Massoumi R, Podda M, Fassler R, et al. Cylindroma as tumor of hair follicle origin. J Invest Dermatol 2006;126(5):1182–4.
3. Ancell H. History of a remarkable case of tumours, developed on the head and face; accompanied with a similar disease in the abdomen. Med Chir Trans 1842;25:227–306.11.
4. Brooke HG. Epithelioma adenoides cysticum. Br J Dermatol 1892;4:268–87.
5. Spiegler E. Ueber endotheliome der haut. Arch Dermatol Res 1899;50(2):163–76.
6. Knudson AG Jr. Mutation and cancer: statistical study of retinoblastoma. Proc Natl Acad Sci U S A 1971;68(4):820–3.
7. Rajan N, Langtry JA, Ashworth A, et al. Tumor mapping in 2 large multigenerational families with CYLD mutations: implications for disease management and tumor induction. Arch Dermatol 2009;145(11):1277–84.
8. Evans CD. Turban tumour. Br J Dermatol 1954;66(12):434–43.
9. Blake PW, Toro JR. Update of cylindromatosis gene (CYLD) mutations in Brooke-Spiegler syndrome: novel insights into the role of deubiquitination in cell signaling. Hum Mutat 2009;30(7):1025–36.
10. van Balkom ID, Hennekam RC. Dermal eccrine cylindromatosis. J Med Genet 1994;31(4):321–4.
11. Sellheyer K. Spiradenoma and cylindroma originate from the hair follicle bulge and not from the eccrine sweat gland: an immunohistochemical study with CD200 and other stem cell markers. J Cutan Pathol 2015;42(2):90–101.
12. Cotton DW, Braye SG. Dermal cylindromas originate from the eccrine sweat gland. Br J Dermatol 1984;111(1):53–61.
13. Bilroth T. Die cylindergeschwulst (cylindroma). Untersuchungenuber die Entwicklung der Blutgefasse, nebstBeobachtungenaus der koniglichenchirugischen Universtats-Klink zu Berlin. Berlin: G Riemer; 1856. p. 55–69.
14. Michal M, Lamovec J, Mukensnabl P, et al. Spiradenocylindromas of the skin: tumors with morphological features of spiradenoma and cylindroma in the same lesion: report of 12 cases. Pathol Int 1999;49(5):419–25.
15. Kazakov DV, Magro G, Kutzner H, et al. Spiradenoma and spiradenocylindroma with an adenomatous or atypical adenomatous component: a clinicopathological study of 6 cases. Am J Dermatopathol 2008;30(5):436–41.
16. Rajan N, Burn J, Langtry J, et al. Transition from cylindroma to spiradenoma in CYLD-defective tumours is associated with reduced DKK2 expression. J Pathol 2011;224(3):309–21.
17. Coulombe PA, Kopan R, Fuchs E. Expression of keratin K14 in the epidermis and hair follicle: insights into complex programs of differentiation. J Cell Biol 1989;109(5):2295–312.
18. Freedman AM, Woods JE. Total scalp excision and auricular resurfacing for dermal cylindroma (turban tumor). Ann Plast Surg 1989;22(1):50–7.
19. Gerretsen AL, van der Putte SC, Deenstra W, et al. Cutaneous cylindroma with malignant transformation. Cancer 1993;72(5):1618–23.

20. Durani BK, Kurzen H, Jaeckel A, et al. Malignant transformation of multiple dermal cylindromas. Br J Dermatol 2001;145(4):653–6.

21. Kazakov DV, Zelger B, Rutten A, et al. Morphologic diversity of malignant neoplasms arising in preexisting spiradenoma, cylindroma, and spiradenocylindroma based on the study of 24 cases, sporadic or occurring in the setting of Brooke-Spiegler syndrome. Am J Surg Pathol 2009;33(5): 705–19.

22. Weedon D. Weedon's skin pathology. 3rd edition. London: Churchill Livingstone Elsevier; 2010.

23. Melly L, Lawton G, Rajan N. Basal cell carcinoma arising in association with trichoepithelioma in a case of Brooke-Spiegler syndrome with a novel genetic mutation in CYLD. J Cutan Pathol 2012; 39(10):977–8.

24. Schulz T, Proske S, Hartschuh W, et al. High-grade trichoblastic carcinoma arising in trichoblastoma: a rare adnexal neoplasm often showing metastatic spread. Am J Dermatopathol 2005;27(1):9–16.

25. Chang YC, Colome-Grimmer M, Kelly E. Multiple trichoepitheliomas in the lines of Blaschko. Pediatr Dermatol 2006;23(2):149–51.

26. Furuichi M, Makino T, Yamakoshi T, et al. Blaschkoid distribution of cylindromas in a germline CYLD mutation carrier. Br J Dermatol 2012;166(6):1376–8.

27. Blaschko A. Die Nevenverteilung in derhant in ihrer Beziehung zuden Ekrankungender Haut. Verhand Deust Dermatol Gessel. 1901.

28. Moss C, Larkins S, Stacey M, et al. Epidermal mosaicism and Blaschko's lines. J Med Genet 1993;30(9): 752–5.

29. Happle R. Segmental forms of autosomal dominant skin disorders: different types of severity reflect different states of zygosity. Am J Med Genet 1996; 66(2):241–2.

30. Jungehulsing M, Wagner M, Damm M. Turban tumour with involvement of the parotid gland. J Laryngol Otol 1999;113(8):779–83.

31. Biggs PJ, Wooster R, Ford D, et al. Familial cylindromatosis (turban tumour syndrome) gene localised to chromosome 16q12-q13: evidence for its role as a tumour suppressor gene. Nat Genet 1995;11(4): 441–3.

32. Bignell GR, Warren W, Seal S, et al. Identification of the familial cylindromatosis tumour-suppressor gene. Nat Genet 2000;25(2):160–5.

33. Takahashi M, Rapley E, Biggs PJ, et al. Linkage and LOH studies in 19 cylindromatosis families show no evidence of genetic heterogeneity and refine the CYLD locus on chromosome 16q12-q13. Hum Genet 2000;106(1):58–65.

34. Zhang XJ, Liang YH, He PP, et al. Identification of the cylindromatosis tumor-suppressor gene responsible for multiple familial trichoepithelioma. J Invest Dermatol 2004;122(3):658–64.

35. Stephens PJ, Davies HR, Mitani Y, et al. Whole exome sequencing of adenoid cystic carcinoma. J Clin Invest 2013;123(7):2965–8.

36. Cunningham F, Amode MR, Barrell D, et al. Ensembl 2015. Nucleic Acids Res 2015;43(Database issue): D662–9.

37. Zuo YG, Xu Y, Wang B, et al. A novel mutation of CYLD in a Chinese family with multiple familial trichoepithelioma and no CYLD protein expression in the tumour tissue. Br J Dermatol 2007;157(4):818–21.

38. Nijman SM, Luna-Vargas MP, Velds A, et al. A genomic and functional inventory of deubiquitinating enzymes. Cell 2005;123(5):773–86.

39. Gao J, Huo L, Sun X, et al. The tumor suppressor CYLD regulates microtubule dynamics and plays a role in cell migration. J Biol Chem 2008;283(14): 8802–9.

40. Massoumi R, Paus R. Cylindromatosis and the CYLD gene: new lessons on the molecular principles of epithelial growth control. Bioessays 2007;29(12): 1203–14.

41. Kloepper JE, Ernst N, Krieger K, et al. NF-kappa B activity is required for anagen maintenance in human hair follicles in vitro. J Invest Dermatol 2014; 134(7):2036–8.

42. Trompouki E, Hatzivassiliou E, Tsichritzis T, et al. CYLD is a deubiquitinating enzyme that negatively regulates NF-kappaB activation by TNFR family members. Nature 2003;424(6950):793–6.

43. Massoumi R. Ubiquitin chain cleavage: CYLD at work. Trends Biochem Sci 2010;35(7):392–9.

44. Reiley WW, Jin W, Lee AJ, et al. Deubiquitinating enzyme CYLD negatively regulates the ubiquitin-dependent kinase Tak1 and prevents abnormal T cell responses. J Exp Med 2007;204(6):1475–85.

45. Massoumi R, Chmielarska K, Hennecke K, et al. Cyld inhibits tumor cell proliferation by blocking Bcl-3-dependent NF-kappaB signaling. Cell 2006; 125(4):665–77.

46. Kovalenko A, Chable-Bessia C, Cantarella G, et al. The tumour suppressor CYLD negatively regulates NF-kappaB signalling by deubiquitination. Nature 2003;424(6950):801–5.

47. Reiley W, Zhang M, Sun SC. Negative regulation of JNK signaling by the tumor suppressor CYLD. J Biol Chem 2004;279(53):55161–7.

48. Tauriello DV, Haegebarth A, Kuper I, et al. Loss of the tumor suppressor CYLD enhances Wnt/beta-catenin signaling through K63-linked ubiquitination of Dvl. Mol Cell 2010;37(5):607–19.

49. Rajan N, Elliott RJ, Smith A, et al. The cylindromatosis gene product, CYLD, interacts with MIB2 to regulate notch signaling. Oncotarget 2014;5(23):12126–40.

50. Lim JH, Jono H, Komatsu K, et al. CYLD negatively regulates transforming growth factor-beta-signalling via deubiquitinating Akt. Nat Commun 2012;3:771.

51. Rajan N, Ashworth A. Inherited cylindromas: lessons from a rare tumour. Lancet. Oncol 2015;16(9):e460–9.

52. Vanecek T, Halbhuber Z, Kacerovska D, et al. Large germline deletions of the CYLD gene in patients with Brooke-Spiegler syndrome and multiple familial trichoepithelioma. Am J Dermatopathol 2014;36(11): 868–74.

53. Nagy N, Farkas K, Kemeny L, et al. Phenotype-genotype correlations for clinical variants caused by CYLD mutations. Eur J Med Genet 2015;58(5):271–8.

54. Poblete Gutierrez P, Eggermann T, Holler D, et al. Phenotype diversity in familial cylindromatosis: a frameshift mutation in the tumor suppressor gene CYLD underlies different tumors of skin appendages. J Invest Dermatol 2002;119(2):527–31.

55. Nagy N, Rajan N, Farkas K, et al. A mutational hotspot in CYLD causing cylindromas: a comparison of phenotypes arising in different genetic backgrounds. Acta Derm Venereol 2013;93(6):743–5.

56. Kazakov DV, Thoma-Uszynski S, Vanecek T, et al. A case of Brooke-Spiegler syndrome with a novel germline deep intronic mutation in the CYLD gene leading to intronic exonization, diverse somatic mutations, and unusual histology. Am J Dermatopathol 2009;31(7):664–73.

57. Massoumi R, Kuphal S, Hellerbrand C, et al. Downregulation of CYLD expression by Snail promotes tumor progression in malignant melanoma. J Exp Med 2009;206(1):221–32.

58. Hellerbrand C, Bumes E, Bataille F, et al. Reduced expression of CYLD in human colon and hepatocellular carcinomas. Carcinogenesis 2007;28(1):21–7.

59. Zhong S, Fields CR, Su N, et al. Pharmacologic inhibition of epigenetic modifications, coupled with gene expression profiling, reveals novel targets of aberrant DNA methylation and histone deacetylation in lung cancer. Oncogene 2007;26(18):2621–34.

60. Annunziata CM, Davis RE, Demchenko Y, et al. Frequent engagement of the classical and alternative NF-kappaB pathways by diverse genetic abnormalities in multiple myeloma. Cancer Cell 2007; 12(2):115–30.

61. Beltran H, Prandi D, Mosquera JM, et al. Divergent clonal evolution of castration-resistant neuroendocrine prostate cancer. Nat Med 2016;22(3): 298–305.

62. Rajan N, Trainer AH, Burn J, et al. Familial cylindromatosis and Brooke-Spiegler syndrome: a review of current therapeutic approaches and the surgical challenges posed by two affected families. Dermatol Surg 2009;35(5):845–52.

63. Oosterkamp HM, Neering H, Nijman SM, et al. An evaluation of the efficacy of topical application of salicylic acid for the treatment of familial cylindromatosis. Br J Dermatol 2006;155(1):182–5.

64. Fisher GH, Geronemus RG. Treatment of multiple familial trichoepitheliomas with a combination of aspirin and a neutralizing antibody to tumor necrosis factor alpha: A case report and hypothesis of mechanism. Arch Dermatol 2006;142(6): 782–3.

65. Martins C, Bartolo E. Brooke-Spiegler syndrome: treatment of cylindromas with CO_2 laser. Dermatol Surg 2000;26(9):877–80 [discussion: 881].

Interleukin-22 and Cyclosporine in Aggressive Cutaneous Squamous Cell Carcinoma

Alexis L. Santana, PhD[a], Diane Felsen, PhD[b],
John A. Carucci, MD, PhD[a],*

KEYWORDS

- Squamous cell carcinoma • Cyclosporine • IL-22 • Organ transplant recipient
- Transplant-associated squamous cell carcinoma • Immunosuppression
- Nonmelanoma skin cancer

KEY POINTS

- Cutaneous squamous cell carcinoma (SCC) is frequently curable, but causes significant morbidity and mortality, particularly in immune-suppressed organ transplant recipients.
- The SCC tumor microenvironment is rich and composed of multiple subsets of immune cells that exert antitumor and protumor effects.
- Interleukin (IL)-22 and its receptor are highly expressed in SCC and more so in transplant-associated SCC.
- IL-22 mediates SCC proliferation; an effect that is potentiated by cyclosporine.
- IL-22 blockade results in decreased SCC burden in a murine model system in vivo and may represent a therapeutic target.

INTRODUCTION

Cutaneous squamous cell carcinoma (SCC) is the second most common human malignancy, with more than 700,000 cases expected in 2016.[1–4] Although typically curable by excision with clear margins, SCC can behave aggressively and metastasize to local lymph nodes despite treatment.[5–7] Cutaneous SCC is characterized by the malignant proliferation of keratinocytes that typically occurs on sun-damaged skin and tends to develop within areas of noninvasive actinic keratosis (AK). Progression from AK to SCC is thought to occur as a result of ultraviolet (UV)-induced mutations in proto-oncogene genes, with as few as 2 mutations being sufficient to drive SCC development.[8,9] Additional factors from the tumor microenvironment likely influence SCC progression.

THE TUMOR MICROENVIRONMENT OF SQUAMOUS CELL CARCINOMA

Gene expression profiling of invasive SCC has revealed the presence of a large inflammatory response.[10] On a broad level, immune cells are thought to play a role in the antitumor response. These immune cells include Langerhans cells

Conflict of Interest: The authors have no conflicts of interest.
[a] The Ronald O. Perelman Department of Dermatology, New York University School of Medicine, 522 First Avenue, New York, NY 10016, USA; [b] Institute for Pediatric Urology, Department of Urology, Weill Cornell Medical College, 1300 York Avenue, Box 94, New York, NY 10065, USA
* Corresponding author. The Ronald O. Perelman Department of Dermatology, New York University School of Medicine, 240 East 38th Street 11th Floor, New York, NY 10016.
E-mail address: john.carucci@nyumc.org

Dermatol Clin 35 (2017) 73–84
http://dx.doi.org/10.1016/j.det.2016.07.003
0733-8635/17/© 2016 Elsevier Inc. All rights reserved.

(LCs), dermal dendritic cells (DCs), CD4+ and CD8+ T cells, T regulatory cells (Treg), macrophages, and natural killer (NK) cells. For SCC, some cell types typically implicated in tumor eradication, NK, B cells, and monocytes, are rarely detected surrounding and infiltrating tumors.[11] However, CD4+ and CD8+ T cells, DCs, and tumor-associated macrophages (TAMs) are often found infiltrating SCC tumors (**Fig. 1**).[11,12] These cells are thought to stunt malignancy and promote regression of primary tumors, but in the context of SCC some of these cell types may be functionally impaired or may exert protumor effects.

T cells are a significant component of the SCC microenvironment.[13–17] Gene expression profiling has shown that T-cell activity is decreased in SCC, as shown by downregulation of activation maker CD69 and impaired secretion of granzyme B and inducible nitric oxide synthase (iNOS).[10] In addition, myeloid-derived suppressor cells are present in SCC and function to impair T cell–mediated immunity by secreting nitric oxide in the tumor microenvironment. The consequence of this is dampening E-selectin expression on epithelial cells and impairment of T-cell entry into tumors.[18] In contrast, human T cells have been reported to secrete interleukin (IL)-24 in response to antigen stimulation, secretion of which has been shown to increase matrix metalloproteinase (MMP)-7 gene expression by SCC cells in culture, potentially contributing to SCC invasion.[19,20] Antibody blocking of SCC cells

with MMP-7–specific antibody has been shown to significantly delay SCC migration.[19]

Antigen-presenting cells (APCs) in the skin include epidermal LCs and dermal myeloid DCs. Myeloid DCs from SCC do not stimulate T-cell proliferation, even when cultured in the presence of maturation promoting cytokines such as IL-1β, IL-6, tumor necrosis factor alpha (TNFα) and prostaglandin E2.[21] These data might indicate a significant gap in defense against SCC. This possibility is further supported by the presence of IL-10 and transforming growth factor beta (TGFβ) in the SCC microenvironment and expression of CD200 receptor by SCC-associated DCs.[21,22] Each of these has been shown to decrease DC-mediated T-cell responses.[23] LCs, located in the epidermal layer, should be the first APCs to encounter SCC tumor antigens generated by transformed keratinocytes. These cells are primarily found in tissues adjacent to and including the interface with the tumor.[24] Moreover, LCs from SCC have been shown to stimulate CD4+ and CD8+ T-cell proliferation at rates higher than those from normal skin eliciting a type 1 T-cell response.[24] In addition, they express higher levels of LC maturation markers, CD40, CD80, CD83, and CD86. This finding might indicate an antitumor role for LCs in human SCC. In contrast, diphtheria toxin depletion of LCs in mice decreases ultraviolet B (UVB)–induced SCC tumor growth.[25] These data suggest that LC responses somehow contribute to SCC tumor growth. LCs from SCC have been reported to express immune-activating signal transducer and activator of transcription (STAT) 4, IL-15, and CD80, and immune tolerizing CD200 genes.[24] Therefore, it is possible that LCs can have protumor roles in the context of SCC, despite their ability to elicit T-cell responses.

An abundance of TAMs are found surrounding as well as penetrating SCC.[26] TAMs may play a dual role in the tumor microenvironment, because they maintain the potential to eradicate tumor cells but have been shown to promote tumor growth. TAMs in the SCC microenvironment have been shown to be classically activated M1 marker, alternatively activated M2 marker, or biactivated M1 and M2 marker expressing (**Fig. 2**).[27,28] M1 activation is driven through the type 1 T helper (Th1) cytokine interferon gamma (IFNγ),[27,29] whereas M2 activation occurs as a result of type 2 T helper (Th2) cytokines, which include IL-10, IL-13, and IL-4.[29] Although M1 macrophage responses are thought to prevent tumor growth, the predominant subtype found in SCC tumors are M2 macrophages, which have lower antigen-processing capacity.[30] In addition, they have been shown to negatively correlate with tumor growth and

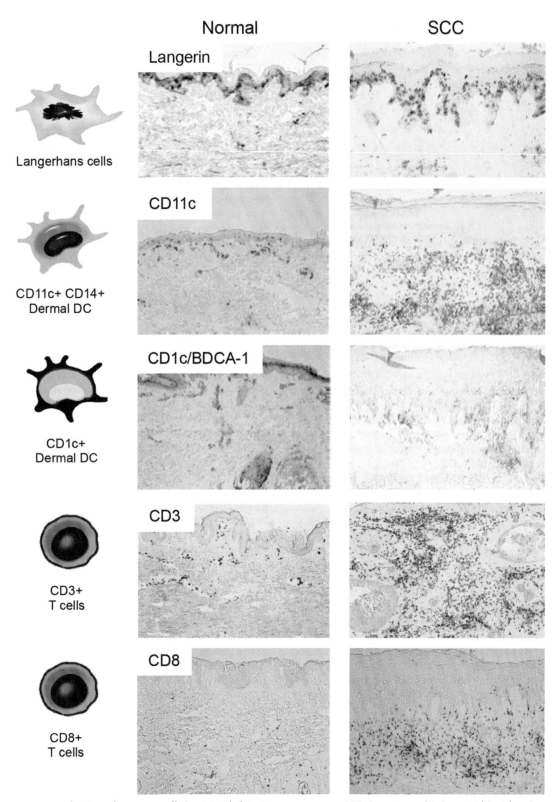

Fig. 1. Distribution of immune cells in normal skin versus cutaneous SCC. Representative immunohistochemistry showing the relative abundance of Langerhans cells (Langerin), Dermal DCs (CD11c+ and CD1c+), and T cells (CD3+ and CD8+). Frozen tissue sections of normal skin and SCCs were stained with the following antibodies:

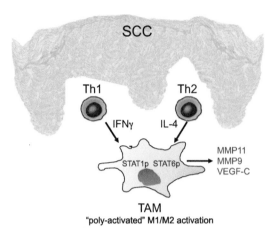

SCC

Th1   Th2

IFNγ   IL-4

STAT1p STAT6p → MMP11
                 MMP9
                 VEGF-C

TAM
"poly-activated" M1/M2 activation

Fig. 2. Model of cutaneous SCC macrophage polarization. Th1 and Th2 cells in the microenvironment produce interferon gamma (IFNγ) and IL-4, respectively. These cytokines stimulate M1 classic and M2 alternative phenotypes, resulting in poly activated TAMs. TAMs are characterized by the presence of phosphorylated STAT1 and STAT6 and expression of MMP-11, MMP-9, and vascular endothelial growth factor C (VEGF-C).

progression. The authors found that SCC TAMs express MMP-11, MMP-9, STAT1, STAT6, and vascular endothelial growth factor C (VEGF-C), which have been shown to promote increased lymphatic vessel density that is correlated with increased metastasis.[31–33] Hence, SCC TAMs may show poor antigen-presentation capacity in addition to secreting factors that may potentiate tumor progression.

TRANSPLANT-ASSOCIATED SQUAMOUS CELL CARCINOMA

Solid organ transplant recipients (OTRs) represent a particularly high-risk population for the development of SCC. Immunosuppressive therapy used by OTRs to prevent allograft rejection predisposes patients to cutaneous infections and neoplasms.[34] OTRs are 60 to 100 times more likely to develop transplant-associated SCC (TSCC) compared with age-matched immune-competent populations.[4,35] Patients with TSCC may experience

catastrophic body surface area involvement with metastatic rates as high as 8% (**Fig. 3**).[3,36–39]

Similar to SCC in immune-competent patients, TSCC tumors were shown to have heightened levels of inflammatory gene expression measured using gene set enrichment analysis.[40] More recently, the authors showed that TSCC tumors contain a higher percentage of IL-22–producing CD8+ T cells and increased expression of the IL-22 receptor.[41] IL-22 has been shown to promote SCC proliferation in a dose-dependent manner in vitro. In addition, IL-22 drives inflammation and suppresses keratinocyte apoptosis; this may explain the increased proliferation and poorer outcomes observed in patients with TSCC.[41,42]

GENERAL OVERVIEW OF INTERLEUKIN-22 SIGNALING

Interleukin (IL) 22 is a cytokine that was discovered in 2000 after being cloned from activated T cells.[43–45] IL-22 targets cell types comprising outer-body barriers such as respiratory and intestinal epithelial cells, hepatocytes, and keratinocytes, but not cells of hematopoietic origin. The cytokine plays an important role in tissue homeostasis, tissue repair, and wound healing.[43] Moreover, its expression has been linked to the development and progression of multiple carcinomas.[46–51]

IL-22 is characterized as an IL-10 cytokine family member along with IL-10, IL-20, IL-24, and IL-26.[43,52,53] The cytokine signals via the heterodimeric transmembrane IL22 receptor (IL-22R) 1 and IL-10R2, and shares IL-22R1 with 2 other IL-10 family members, IL-20 and IL-24.[45,54] Signaling through the IL-22 receptor primarily induces Janus kinase activity and STAT transcription factors. In primary cells, STAT3 activation is the main event observed, along with weak activation of STAT1 and/or STAT5.[53] In addition, activation of mitogen-activated protein kinase (MAPK), phosphoinositide 3-kinase (PI3K), and AKT–mammalian target of rapamycin (mTOR) also occurs.[42,55–59]

The cellular sources of IL-22 are CD4+ T cells (Th17, Th22), CD8+ T cells (Tc17, Tc22), γδ T cells, NK T cells, and lymphoid tissue inducer cells.[60,61] Although a wide variety of innate and

Langerin (Immunotech), CD11C (BD Pharmigen), CD1C/BDCA-1 (Biosource), and CD3 and CD8 (BD Pharmingen). Biotin-labeled horse anti-mouse antibody (Vector Laboratories) was then amplified with avidin-biotin complex (Vector Laboratories) and developed with a chromogen 3-amino-9-ethylcarbazole (Sigma Aldrich). Counterstaining was then carried out with light green (Sigma-Aldrich). With each immunohistochemistry experiment the appropriate isotype controls were performed. (10× magnification). (*Adapted from* Yanofsky VR, Mitsui H, Felsen D, et al. Understanding dendritic cells and their role in cutaneous carcinoma and cancer immunotherapy. Clin Dev Immunol 2013;2013:624123; and Zhang S, Fujita H, Mitsui H, et al. Increased Tc22 and Treg/CD8 ratio contribute to aggressive growth of transplant associated squamous cell carcinoma. PLoS One 2013;8(5):e62154; with permission.)

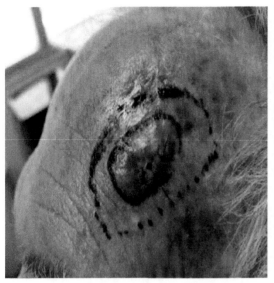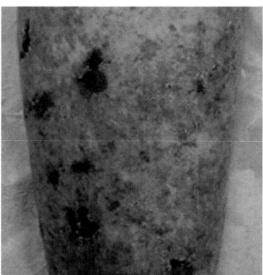

Fig. 3. TSCC. In transit metastatic SCC is defined by the presence of dermal or subcutaneous papules or nodules that occur between the site of the primary tumor and lymph node basin. This patient (*left*) presented with in transit metastases 6 weeks after resection of a high-risk, primary SCC. Some patients with catastrophic carcinomatosis develop extensive field disease with confluent AK, in situ SCCs involving more than 50% body surface area (*right*). (*From* Belkin D, Carucci JA. Mohs surgery for squamous cell carcinoma. Dermatol Clin 2011;29(2):169; with permission.)

adaptive cell types have been shown to secrete IL-22, CD4+ T cells (Th17 and Th22) and innate lymphoid cells are considered the predominant source of IL-22 in humans. As mentioned earlier, CD4+ and CD8+ T cells, often found infiltrating tumors, play an important role in SCC progression.[11]

ROLE OF INTERLEUKIN-22 IN SQUAMOUS CELL CARCINOMA

The role of IL-22 in skin cancer is an area of active research. It was reported that cutaneous SCCs contain high numbers of infiltrating IL-22–producing CD4+ T cells, whose recruitment to the tumor partially depended on matrix metalloproteinase 10 (MMP-10) and S100A15 production.[62] The authors found IL-22, IL-22R, and downstream mediator phosphorylated STAT3 (pSTAT3) to be highly expressed in SCC (**Fig. 4**).[41] Further, IL-22 treatment of SCC results in enhanced proliferation in vitro (**Fig. 5**).[41] IL-22 has been shown to increase iNOS expression and activity, contributing to proinflammatory as well as proangiogenic properties in colon carcinoma cells.[51] In SCC, iNOS expression has been reported and correlates with enhanced tumorigenic potential.[63,64] SCC-associated DCs contain a subset of TNFα-positive, iNOS-positive cells.[21] Dermal keratinocyte iNOS expression is enhanced by UVB irradiation, which is an environmental factor linked to SCC development.[65–69] Further studies are necessary to determine

whether IL-22 treatment coupled with UVB irradiation could promote increased SCC tumor growth as a result of iNOS expression. Importantly, administration of IL-22 antibody to SKH-1 animals during UVB-induced cutaneous carcinoma resulted in a decrease in the number and size of SCC tumors.[70] This result further confirms the role of IL-22 in promoting SCC tumorigenesis.

CHANGES IN THE SQUAMOUS CELL CARCINOMA TUMOR MICROENVIRONMENT INFLUENCED BY CYCLOSPORINE A

OTRs require immune-suppressive drugs to prevent allograft rejection. These drugs include cyclosporine A (CSA), which was considered the mainstay of therapy until recently. CSA prevents T-cell activation by binding cyclophilin molecules, which are needed for calcineurin phosphatase activity. Calcineurin phosphatase activity induces nuclear factor of activated T cell (NFAT) transcription of immune-related cytokine genes, such as IL-2 and IFNγ, expression of which is detrimental to allograft maintenance in OTRs.[71–73]

Effects of Cyclosporine A on Immune Cell Infiltrates

Differences in immune infiltrates are found in SCC compared with TSCC tumors and have revealed a shift in the microenvironment that favors tumor

Normal   SCC   TSCC

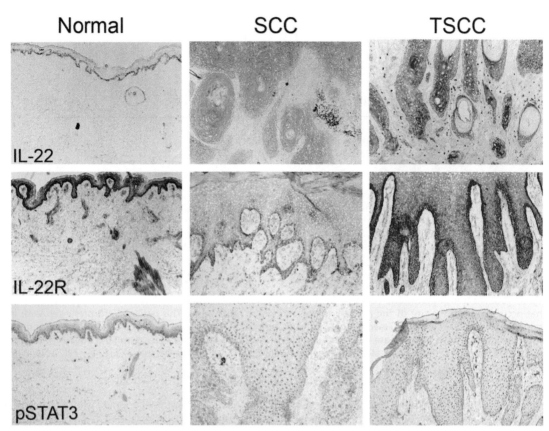

Fig. 4. IL-22 cytokine, receptor, and downstream signaling is enhanced in TSCC. Immunohistochemistry performed on normal, SCC and TSCC shows enhanced expression of IL-22, IL-22R, and pSTAT3. Frozen tissue sections of normal skin and SCCs and TSCCs were stained with the following antibodies: IL-22 (R&D systems), IL-22 Receptor (Prosci), and pSTAT3 (Santa Cruz Biotechnology). Biotin-labeled horse anti-mouse antibody (Vector Laboratories) was then amplified with avidin-biotin complex (Vector Laboratories) and developed with a chromogen 3-amino-9-ethylcarbazole (Sigma Aldrich). Counterstaining was then carried out with light green (Sigma-Aldrich). With each immunohistochemistry experiment the appropriate isotype controls were performed. (10× magnification). (*Adapted from* Zhang S, Fujita H, Mitsui H, et al. Increased Tc22 and Treg/CD8 ratio contribute to aggressive growth of transplant associated squamous cell carcinoma. PLoS One 2013;8(5):e62154; with permission.)

occurrence and malignancy. The authors have shown that TSCCs have an increased ratio of Treg to cytotoxic CD8+ T cells and a lower percentage of IFNγ-producing CD4+ T cells compared with immune-competent SCC.[41] In addition, the Tregs are immune-suppressive cells that are present at a higher proportion in TSCC tumors and may contribute to poor prognosis by suppressing antitumor activity and aiding in immune evasion.[74–76] CD4+ helper T cells infiltrating TSCC tumors are reduced for IL17A mRNA, a Th17-specific cytokine involved in inflammation that promotes recruitment of innate immune cells.[41,77,78]

CD8+ T cells producing IFNγ play an important role in combatting aggressive tumor behavior and were shown to be decreased in TSCC compared with SCC.[41] Despite decreased proportions of CD8+ T-cell infiltrate, there was an increase in

the Tc22 polarization in TSCC tumors.[41] The levels of IL-22 cytokine, IL-22R, and phosphorylated STAT3 were dramatically increased in TSCC compared with SCC (see **Fig. 4**).[41] Treatment of peripheral blood mononuclear cell (PBMC)-derived T cells from healthy volunteers cultured with CSA resulted in a decrease in the number of CD4+ and CD8+ IFNγ-producing and IL-17–producing cells but had no effect on those producing IL-4 and IL-22.[70] As a result, CSA treatment increases the proportion of T22 cells compared with other T-cell subtypes.

Effects of Cyclosporine A on Squamous Cell Carcinoma

CSA has been implicated in promoting SCC. For instance, CSA treatment has been shown to

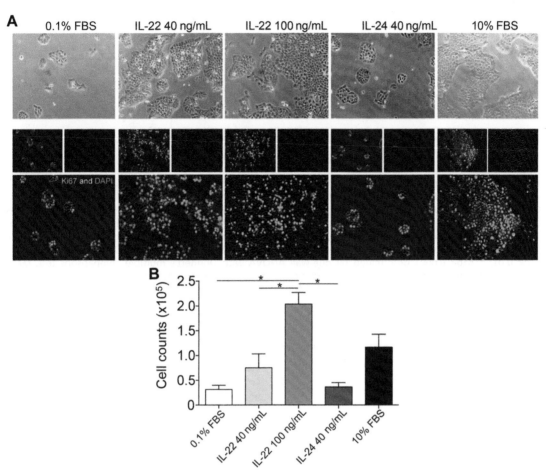

Fig. 5. IL-22 treatment enhances human cutaneous SCC proliferation. (*A*) A431 cells were cultured in 0.1% fetal bovine serum (FBS) serum starvation conditions with or without the indicated cytokines for 72 hours. Cells cultured in the presence of IL-22 cytokine or 10% FBS showed increased colony formation compared with those grown under serum starvation conditions or treated with IL-24. The phase images (*below*) are representative immunofluorescence images staining for the Ki-67 proliferation marker (*green*) and nuclear 4,6-diamidino-2-phenylindole (DAPI) (*blue*). (*B*) Cell counts were performed after 72 hours in the indicated conditions and show enhanced cell numbers after treatment with control 10% FBS and IL-22 conditions (1-way analysis of variance [ANOVA], $P<.001$). *$p< 0.05$, determined by one-way ANOVA. (*From* Zhang S, Fujita H, Mitsui H, et al. Increased Tc22 and Treg/CD8 ratio contribute to aggressive growth of transplant associated squamous cell carcinoma. PLoS One 2013;8(5):e62154; with permission.)

induce phenotypic changes in SCC cells by promoting tumor growth and increasing invasive potential.[79,80] CSA treatment was shown to counteract p53-dependent SCC tumor cell senescence, thereby increasing tumorigenesis.[80] In addition, CSA treatment of nude mice, which lack a functional immune system, has been shown to promote the growth of SCC keratinocytes in vivo.[81] Moreover, CSA treatment inhibits keratinocyte UVB-induced DNA damage repair and apoptosis by inhibiting NFAT expression.[82] CSA is a calcineurin inhibitor that inhibits NFAT expression, a transcription factor that has been shown to promote phosphatase and tensin homolog (PTEN) transcription.[83] UV-irradiated keratinocyte growth and survival were increased by CSA treatment through enhancement of AKT activation by suppressing PTEN transcription.[81] The mechanism by which CSA inhibits PTEN transcription to promote keratinocyte survival is unknown, because there are no canonical NFAT binding sites in the PTEN promoter. In addition, CSA enhanced IL-22 promotion of SCC growth, resulting in increased cell proliferation, enhanced colony formation, and increased cell numbers (Fig. 6).[70] Moreover, CSA and IL-22, alone or in combination, enhanced SCC migratory and invasive potential in vitro.[70]

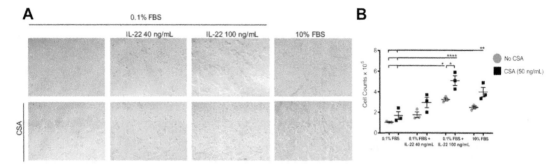

Fig. 6. Cyclosporine treatment potentiates IL-22–mediated human cutaneous SCC proliferation. (*A*) A431 cells were cultured in 0.1% FBS serum starvation conditions with or without the indicated cytokines for 72 hours. CSA treatment increased growth and colony formation either alone in serum starvation conditions or in the presence of IL-22 cytokine or 10% FBS. (*B*) Cell counts performed on A431 cells treated in the indicated conditions. CSA treatment increased proliferation alone, in serum starvation conditions, or in the presence of IL-22 cytokine. Data are representative of 3 experiments ± standard error of the mean (1-way ANOVA, $P<.001$). *$p< 0.05$, **$p< 0.01$, ****$p< 0.0001$ determined by one-way ANOVA with Dunnett's multiple comparisons test. (*From* Abikhair M, Mitsui H, Yanofsky V, et al. Cyclosporine A immunosuppression drives catastrophic squamous cell carcinoma through IL-22. JCI Insight 2016;1(8):e86434; with permission.)

SUMMARY

CSA is an immunosuppressive agent widely used to support organ transplant. Until recently, immunosuppression was considered the mechanism by which CSA causes SCC. However, recent studies suggest that CSA treatment favors malignant progression in more ways than previously thought. First, CSA treatment had been shown to increase SCC tumor growth in mice that have no immune system for CSA to suppress.[81] CSA functions to enhance the survival and growth of

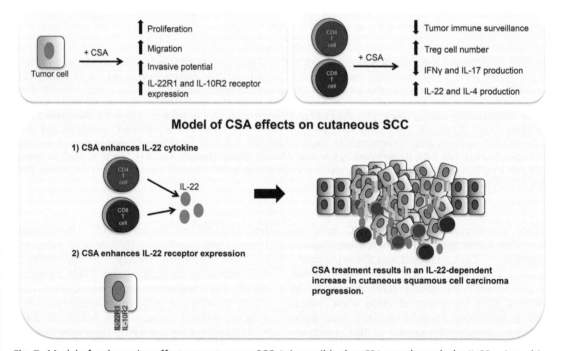

Fig. 7. Model of cyclosporine effects on cutaneous SCC. It is possible that CSA acts through the IL-22 axis to drive aggressive behavior by SCC. CSA treatment promotes SCC growth, invasive capacity, and IL-22 receptor expression. The authors have previously shown that IL-22 treatment promotes SCC growth. In addition to decreased tumor immune surveillance, CSA treatment enhances Treg numbers and IL-22 production by CD4+ and CD8+ T cells. Therefore, higher IL-22 receptor expression on SCC tumor cells and increased levels of IL-22 cytokine produced by CD8+ and CD4+ T cells may contribute to tumor growth.

transformed keratinocytes, even promoting invasive capacity.[79,80] Mechanistic investigations have shown that CSA treatment reduces PTEN transcription, resulting in enhanced AKT activity and cell survival that depends on mTOR signaling. Further delineating the mechanism by which CSA promotes keratinocyte invasive potential and growth may provide insight into the mechanisms of SCC metastasis. Importantly, CSA treatment modulates the repertoire of immune cells in the SCC tumor microenvironment, promoting increased numbers of IL-22–producing immune infiltrates, and treatment of PBMCs with CSA results in enhanced IL-22 production from CD4+ and CD8+ T cells.[70] Because IL-22 has been shown to promote SCC cell growth, migration, and proinflammatory cytokine release, enhanced amounts of IL-22 in the tumor microenvironment of CSA-treated patients could have negative effects (**Fig. 7**). It is possible that CSA acts through the IL-22 axis to drive aggressive behavior by SCC. Further elucidation of the IL-22 axis and its effects on SCC proliferation, migration, and invasion may provide novel rational targets for therapeutic intervention.

REFERENCES

1. Karia PS, Han J, Schmults CD. Cutaneous squamous cell carcinoma: estimated incidence of disease, nodal metastasis, and deaths from disease in the United States, 2012. J Am Acad Dermatol 2013;68(6):957–66.

2. Weinberg AS, Ogle CA, Shim EK. Metastatic cutaneous squamous cell carcinoma: an update. Dermatol Surg 2007;33(8):885–99.

3. Berg D, Otley CC. Skin cancer in organ transplant recipients: Epidemiology, pathogenesis, and management. J Am Acad Dermatol 2002;47(1):1–17 [quiz: 18–20].

4. Lindelof B, Sigurgeirsson B, Gabel H, et al. Incidence of skin cancer in 5356 patients following organ transplantation. Br J Dermatol 2000;143(3):513–9.

5. Brantsch KD, Meisner C, Schonfisch B, et al. Analysis of risk factors determining prognosis of cutaneous squamous-cell carcinoma: a prospective study. Lancet Oncol 2008;9(8):713–20.

6. Czarnecki D, Staples M, Mar A, et al. Metastases from squamous cell carcinoma of the skin in southern Australia. Dermatology 1994;189(1):52–4.

7. Samarasinghe V, Madan V. Nonmelanoma skin cancer. J Cutan Aesthet Surg 2012;5(1):3–10.

8. Dajee M, Lazarov M, Zhang JY, et al. NF-kappaB blockade and oncogenic Ras trigger invasive human epidermal neoplasia. Nature 2003;421(6923):639–43.

9. Lazarov M, Kubo Y, Cai T, et al. CDK4 coexpression with Ras generates malignant human epidermal tumorigenesis. Nat Med 2002;8(10):1105–14.

10. Haider AS, Peters SB, Kaporis H, et al. Genomic analysis defines a cancer-specific gene expression signature for human squamous cell carcinoma and distinguishes malignant hyperproliferation from benign hyperplasia. J Invest Dermatol 2006;126(4):869–81.

11. Terao H, Nakayama J, Urabe A, et al. Immunohistochemical characterization of cellular infiltrates in squamous cell carcinoma and Bowen's disease occurring in one patient. J Dermatol 1992;19(7):408–13.

12. Yanofsky VR, Mitsui H, Felsen D, et al. Understanding dendritic cells and their role in cutaneous carcinoma and cancer immunotherapy. Clin Dev Immunol 2013;2013:624123.

13. Cho Y, Miyamoto M, Kato K, et al. CD4+ and CD8+ T cells cooperate to improve prognosis of patients with esophageal squamous cell carcinoma. Cancer Res 2003;63(7):1555–9.

14. Claudatus JC Jr, d'Ovidio R, Lospalluti M, et al. Skin tumors and reactive cellular infiltrate: further studies. Acta Derm Venereol 1986;66(1):29–34.

15. De Panfilis G, Colli V, Manfredi G, et al. In situ identification of mononuclear cells infiltrating cutaneous carcinoma: an immuno-histochemical study. Acta Derm Venereol 1979;59(3):219–22.

16. Gatter KC, Morris HB, Roach B, et al. Langerhans' cells and T cells in human skin tumours: an immunohistological study. Histopathology 1984;8(2):229–44.

17. Sznurkowski JJ, Zawrocki A, Emerich J, et al. Prognostic significance of CD4+ and CD8+ T cell infiltration within cancer cell nests in vulvar squamous cell carcinoma. Int J Gynecol Cancer 2011;21(4):717–21.

18. Gehad AE, Lichtman MK, Schmults CD, et al. Nitric oxide-producing myeloid-derived suppressor cells inhibit vascular E-selectin expression in human squamous cell carcinomas. J Invest Dermatol 2012;132(11):2642–51.

19. Mitsui H, Suarez-Farinas M, Gulati N, et al. Gene expression profiling of the leading edge of cutaneous squamous cell carcinoma: IL-24-driven MMP-7. J Invest Dermatol 2014;134(5):1418–27.

20. Poindexter NJ, Walch ET, Chada S, et al. Cytokine induction of interleukin-24 in human peripheral blood mononuclear cells. J Leukoc Biol 2005;78(3):745–52.

21. Bluth MJ, Zaba LC, Moussai D, et al. Myeloid dendritic cells from human cutaneous squamous cell carcinoma are poor stimulators of T-cell proliferation. J Invest Dermatol 2009;129(10):2451–62.

22. Belkin DA, Mitsui H, Wang CQ, et al. CD200 upregulation in vascular endothelium surrounding cutaneous squamous cell carcinoma. JAMA Dermatol 2013;149(2):178–86.

23. Wallet MA, Sen P, Tisch R. Immunoregulation of dendritic cells. Clin Med Res 2005;3(3):166–75.

24. Fujita H, Suarez-Farinas M, Mitsui H, et al. Langerhans cells from human cutaneous squamous cell carcinoma induce strong type 1 immunity. J Invest Dermatol 2012;132(6):1645–55.

25. Lewis JM, Burgler CD, Freudzon M, et al. Langerhans cells facilitate UVB-Induced epidermal carcinogenesis. J Invest Dermatol 2015;135(11):2824–33.

26. Pettersen JS, Fuentes-Duculan J, Suarez-Farinas M, et al. Tumor-associated macrophages in the cutaneous SCC microenvironment are heterogeneously activated. J Invest Dermatol 2011; 131(6):1322–30.

27. Mantovani A, Sica A, Sozzani S, et al. The chemokine system in diverse forms of macrophage activation and polarization. Trends Immunol 2004;25(12): 677–86.

28. Mosser DM, Edwards JP. Exploring the full spectrum of macrophage activation. Nat Rev Immunol 2008; 8(12):958–69.

29. Romagnani S. T-cell subsets (Th1 versus Th2). Ann Allergy Asthma Immunol 2000;85(1):9–18 [quiz 18, 21].

30. Allavena P, Sica A, Garlanda C, et al. The Yin-Yang of tumor-associated macrophages in neoplastic progression and immune surveillance. Immunol Rev 2008;222:155–61.

31. Boone B, Blokx W, De Bacquer D, et al. The role of VEGF-C staining in predicting regional metastasis in melanoma. Virchows Arch 2008;453(3):257–65.

32. Moussai D, Mitsui H, Pettersen JS, et al. The human cutaneous squamous cell carcinoma microenvironment is characterized by increased lymphatic density and enhanced expression of macrophage-derived VEGF-C. J Invest Dermatol 2011;131(1): 229–36.

33. Sugiura T, Inoue Y, Matsuki R, et al. VEGF-C and VEGF-D expression is correlated with lymphatic vessel density and lymph node metastasis in oral squamous cell carcinoma: implications for use as a prognostic marker. Int J Oncol 2009;34(3):673–80.

34. Euvrard S, Kanitakis J, Claudy A. Skin cancers after organ transplantation. N Engl J Med 2003;348(17): 1681–91.

35. Gerlini G, Romagnoli P, Pimpinelli N. Skin cancer and immunosuppression. Crit Rev Oncol Hematol 2005;56(1):127–36.

36. Belkin D, Carucci JA. Mohs surgery for squamous cell carcinoma. Dermatol Clin 2011;29(2):161–74, vii.

37. Campo E, Swerdlow SH, Harris NL, et al. The 2008 WHO classification of lymphoid neoplasms and beyond: evolving concepts and practical applications. Blood 2011;117(19):5019–32.

38. Carucci JA. Cutaneous oncology in organ transplant recipients: meeting the challenge of squamous cell carcinoma. J Invest Dermatol 2004; 123(5):809–16.

39. Ong CS, Keogh AM, Kossard S, et al. Skin cancer in Australian heart transplant recipients. J Am Acad Dermatol 1999;40(1):27–34.

40. Kosmidis M, Dziunycz P, Suarez-Farinas M, et al. Immunosuppression affects CD4+ mRNA expression and induces Th2 dominance in the microenvironment of cutaneous squamous cell carcinoma in organ transplant recipients. J Immunother 2010; 33(5):538–46.

41. Zhang S, Fujita H, Mitsui H, et al. Increased Tc22 and Treg/CD8 ratio contribute to aggressive growth of transplant associated squamous cell carcinoma. PLoS One 2013;8(5):e62154.

42. Wolk K, Witte E, Wallace E, et al. IL-22 regulates the expression of genes responsible for antimicrobial defense, cellular differentiation, and mobility in keratinocytes: a potential role in psoriasis. Eur J Immunol 2006;36(5):1309–23.

43. Dumoutier L, Louahed J, Renauld JC. Cloning and characterization of IL-10-related T cell-derived inducible factor (IL-TIF), a novel cytokine structurally related to IL-10 and inducible by IL-9. J Immunol 2000;164(4):1814–9.

44. Dumoutier L, Van Roost E, Colau D, et al. Human interleukin-10-related T cell-derived inducible factor: molecular cloning and functional characterization as an hepatocyte-stimulating factor. Proc Natl Acad Sci U S A 2000;97(18):10144–9.

45. Xie MH, Aggarwal S, Ho WH, et al. Interleukin (IL)-22, a novel human cytokine that signals through the interferon receptor-related proteins CRF2-4 and IL-22R. J Biol Chem 2000;275(40):31335–9.

46. Kim MJ, Jang JW, Oh BS, et al. Change in inflammatory cytokine profiles after transarterial chemotherapy in patients with hepatocellular carcinoma. Cytokine 2013;64(2):516–22.

47. Qin S, Ma S, Huang X, et al. Th22 cells are associated with hepatocellular carcinoma development and progression. Chin J Cancer Res 2014;26(2): 135–41.

48. Souza JM, Matias BF, Rodrigues CM, et al. IL-17 and IL-22 serum cytokine levels in patients with squamous intraepithelial lesion and invasive cervical carcinoma. Eur J Gynaecol Oncol 2013;34(5): 466–8.

49. Wen Z, Liao Q, Zhao J, et al. High expression of interleukin-22 and its receptor predicts poor prognosis in pancreatic ductal adenocarcinoma. Ann Surg Oncol 2014;21(1):125–32.

50. Zhang W, Chen Y, Wei H, et al. Antiapoptotic activity of autocrine interleukin-22 and therapeutic effects of interleukin-22-small interfering RNA on human lung cancer xenografts. Clin Cancer Res 2008;14(20): 6432–9.

51. Ziesche E, Bachmann M, Kleinert H, et al. The interleukin-22/STAT3 pathway potentiates expression of inducible nitric-oxide synthase in human

colon carcinoma cells. J Biol Chem 2007;282(22): 16006–15.

52. Ouyang W, Rutz S, Crellin NK, et al. Regulation and functions of the IL-10 family of cytokines in inflammation and disease. Annu Rev Immunol 2011;29:71–109.

53. Wolk K, Kunz S, Witte E, et al. IL-22 increases the innate immunity of tissues. Immunity 2004;21(2): 241–54.

54. Kotenko SV, Izotova LS, Mirochnitchenko OV, et al. Identification of the functional interleukin-22 (IL-22) receptor complex: the IL-10R2 chain (IL-10Rbeta) is a common chain of both the IL-10 and IL-22 (IL-10-related T cell-derived inducible factor, IL-TIF) receptor complexes. J Biol Chem 2001; 276(4):2725–32.

55. Andoh A, Zhang Z, Inatomi O, et al. Interleukin-22, a member of the IL-10 subfamily, induces inflammatory responses in colonic subepithelial myofibroblasts. Gastroenterology 2005;129(3):969–84.

56. Ikeuchi H, Kuroiwa T, Hiramatsu N, et al. Expression of interleukin-22 in rheumatoid arthritis: potential role as a proinflammatory cytokine. Arthritis Rheum 2005;52(4):1037–46.

57. Lejeune D, Dumoutier L, Constantinescu S, et al. Interleukin-22 (IL-22) activates the JAK/STAT, ERK, JNK, and p38 MAP kinase pathways in a rat hepatoma cell line. Pathways that are shared with and distinct from IL-10. J Biol Chem 2002;277(37):33676–82.

58. Mitra A, Raychaudhuri SK, Raychaudhuri SP. IL-22 induced cell proliferation is regulated by PI3K/Akt/mTOR signaling cascade. Cytokine 2012;60(1): 38–42.

59. Zhu X, Li Z, Pan W, et al. Participation of Gab1 and Gab2 in IL-22-mediated keratinocyte proliferation, migration, and differentiation. Mol Cell Biochem 2012;369(1–2):255–66.

60. Rutz S, Eidenschenk C, Ouyang W. IL-22, not simply a Th17 cytokine. Immunol Rev 2013;252(1):116–32.

61. Wolk K, Kunz S, Asadullah K, et al. Cutting edge: immune cells as sources and targets of the IL-10 family members? J Immunol 2002;168(11):5397–402.

62. Briso EM, Guinea-Viniegra J, Bakiri L, et al. Inflammation-mediated skin tumorigenesis induced by epidermal c-Fos. Genes Dev 2013;27(18):1959–73.

63. Chen YK, Hsue SS, Lin LM. Increased expression of inducible nitric oxide synthase for human buccal squamous-cell carcinomas: immunohistochemical, reverse transcription-polymerase chain reaction (RT-PCR) and in situ RT-PCR studies. Head Neck 2002;24(10):925–32.

64. Connelly ST, Macabeo-Ong M, Dekker N, et al. Increased nitric oxide levels and iNOS overexpression in oral squamous cell carcinoma. Oral Oncol 2005;41(3):261–7.

65. Baudouin JE, Tachon P. Constitutive nitric oxide synthase is present in normal human keratinocytes. J Invest Dermatol 1996;106(3):428–31.

66. Chang HR, Tsao DA, Wang SR, et al. Expression of nitric oxide synthases in keratinocytes after UVB irradiation. Arch Dermatol Res 2003;295(7):293–6.

67. Sasaki M, Yamaoka J, Miyachi Y. The effect of ultraviolet B irradiation on nitric oxide synthase expression in murine keratinocytes. Exp Dermatol 2000; 9(6):417–22.

68. Seo SJ, Choi HG, Chung HJ, et al. Time course of expression of mRNA of inducible nitric oxide synthase and generation of nitric oxide by ultraviolet B in keratinocyte cell lines. Br J Dermatol 2002;147(4):655–62.

69. Shimizu Y, Sakai M, Umemura Y, et al. Immunohistochemical localization of nitric oxide synthase in normal human skin: expression of endothelial-type and inducible-type nitric oxide synthase in keratinocytes. J Dermatol 1997;24(2):80–7.

70. Abikhair M, Mitsui H, Yanofsky V, et al. Cyclosporine A immunosuppression drives catastrophic squamous cell carcinoma through IL-22. JCI Insight 2016;1(8): 1–12.

71. Granelli-Piperno A. In situ hybridization for interleukin 2 and interleukin 2 receptor mRNA in T cells activated in the presence or absence of cyclosporin A. J Exp Med 1988;168(5):1649–58.

72. Herold KC, Lancki DW, Moldwin RL, et al. Immunosuppressive effects of cyclosporin A on cloned T cells. J Immunol 1986;136(4):1315–21.

73. Kronke M, Leonard WJ, Depper JM, et al. Cyclosporin A inhibits T-cell growth factor gene expression at the level of mRNA transcription. Proc Natl Acad Sci U S A 1984;81(16):5214–8.

74. Beyer M, Kochanek M, Giese T, et al. In vivo peripheral expansion of naive CD4+CD25high FoxP3+ regulatory T cells in patients with multiple myeloma. Blood 2006;107(10):3940–9.

75. Mougiakakos D, Choudhury A, Lladser A, et al. Regulatory T cells in cancer. Adv Cancer Res 2010;107: 57–117.

76. Rutella S, Lemoli RM. Regulatory T cells and tolerogenic dendritic cells: from basic biology to clinical applications. Immunol Lett 2004;94(1–2):11–26.

77. Oukka M. Th17 cells in immunity and autoimmunity. Ann Rheum Dis 2008;67(Suppl 3):iii26–9.

78. Wilson NJ, Boniface K, Chan JR, et al. Development, cytokine profile and function of human interleukin 17-producing helper T cells. Nat Immunol 2007; 8(9):950–7.

79. Hojo M, Morimoto T, Maluccio M, et al. Cyclosporine induces cancer progression by a cell-autonomous mechanism. Nature 1999;397(6719):530–4.

80. Wu X, Nguyen BC, Dziunycz P, et al. Opposing roles for calcineurin and ATF3 in squamous skin cancer. Nature 2010;465(7296):368–72.

81. Han W, Ming M, He TC, et al. Immunosuppressive cyclosporin A activates AKT in keratinocytes through PTEN suppression: implications in skin carcinogenesis. J Biol Chem 2010;285(15):11369–77.

82. Yarosh DB, Pena AV, Nay SL, et al. Calcineurin inhibitors decrease DNA repair and apoptosis in human keratinocytes following ultraviolet B irradiation. J Invest Dermatol 2005;125(5):1020–5.

83. Wang Q, Zhou Y, Jackson LN, et al. Nuclear factor of activated T cells (NFAT) signaling regulates PTEN expression and intestinal cell differentiation. Mol Biol Cell 2011;22(3):412–20.

Melanocytic Nevi and the Genetic and Epigenetic Control of Oncogene-Induced Senescence

Jennifer M. Huang, PhD[a], Ijeuru Chikeka, MD[a],
Thomas J. Hornyak, MD, PhD[a,b,c,*]

KEYWORDS

- Melanocyte • Melanoma • Nevi • Oncogene • Senescence

KEY POINTS

- Melanocytic nevi share oncogenic molecular mutations with melanomas.
- Oncogene-induced senescence explains in part why most nevi are stable and do not undergo progression to malignant melanoma.
- Determining mechanisms that reverse melanoma cells to a senescent phenotype could lead to the identification of therapeutic adjuncts in advanced melanoma.

MELANOCYTIC NEVI

A melanocytic nevus is a benign clonal proliferation of melanocytes, the pigment-producing cells of the epidermis, hair follicle, and uveal tract of the eye.[1] Melanocytes are normally interspersed as single cells among keratinocytes in human skin, resting atop the basement membrane. In melanocytic nevi, they are present in greater concentrations, either singly or in adherent nests or clusters of 3 of more melanocytic cells. The clinical appearances of melanocytic nevi are heterogeneous, associated in part with when during life the nevus is acquired and probably also due to the specific differentiation state of the cell of origin

and their acquired genetic mutations (see later discussion). They can be considered in 2 major groups: congenital and acquired melanocytic nevi.

A congenital nevus is present in 1% to 3% of neonates at birth and shortly thereafter.[2] They are categorized according to their size (small <1.5 cm, medium 1.5–20 cm, large >20 cm– 40 cm, giant>40 cm).[3] Congenital nevi tend to have a globular pattern on dermoscopy and terminal hair follicles. Histologically, congenital nevi consist of big melanocytes that are fusiform, epithelioid, balloon, or neuroid in shape, tracking down from large nests between collagen bundles along cutaneous appendages, vessels, and nerves.[1] They extend deep into the reticular dermis and the subcutis. It

This work was support in part by Merit Review Award 1I01BX002582 from the United States (US) Department of Veterans Affairs, Biomedical Laboratory Research and Development Service; and by National Institutes of Health (NIH) Award R01 AR064810, US Department of Health and Human Services. The contents do not represent the views of the US Department of Veterans Affairs, the US Department of Health and Human Services, or the US government.
[a] Department of Biochemistry and Molecular Biology, University of Maryland School of Medicine, 108 N. Greene St., Baltimore, MD 21201, USA; [b] Research & Development Service, VA Maryland Health Care System, Baltimore, MD, 21201, USA; [c] Department of Dermatology, University of Maryland School of Medicine, Baltimore, MD 21201, USA
* Corresponding author. Department of Biochemistry and Molecular Biology, University of Maryland School of Medicine, 108 N. Greene St., Baltimore, MD 21201.
E-mail address: THornyak@som.umaryland.edu

Dermatol Clin 35 (2017) 85–93
http://dx.doi.org/10.1016/j.det.2016.08.001
0733-8635/17/Published by Elsevier Inc

Abbreviations and acronyms	
ANRIL	Antisense noncoding RNA that is involved in chromatin remodeling, transcription, and post-transcriptional processing. It is often abnormally expressed in cancer.
Atg7	Essential autophagy gene, autophagy-related-7, promotes melanoma by limiting oxidative stress and overcoming senescence; inhibition may be of therapeutic value.
Bmi-1	Polycomb complex protein, member of PRC1, which regulates cell cycle inhibitor genes (p16). Its overexpression may promote tumor invasion and metastasis.
BMP (bone morphogenic protein)	Member of the transforming growth factor-beta (TGF-beta) superfamily that are involved in proliferation, apoptosis, differentiation, chemotaxis, and angiogenesis. It has been shown to have potent antitumor activity in the skin. In melanoma, it is overexpressed and is thought to promote cell invasion and migration.
BMP-Smad1	This signal and its regulation by epigenetic alterations are significant in Ras-induced senescence
BRAF	A member of the RAF family of serine/threonine-specific kinases that is frequently mutated in human melanoma and is a molecular target for therapy
BRAF^{V600E}	The V600E mutation results in an amino acid substitution of valine (V) to glutamic acid (E) at position 600 of BRAF.
EED (embryonic ectoderm development)	Component of PRC2
EZH2 (enhancer of zeste homolog 2)	Epigenetic modifier and catalytic component of the polycomb repressive complex 2 (PRC2), which is thought to promote growth and metastasis of melanoma. Increased expression is associated with uncontrolled proliferation in melanoma.
HRAS^{G12V}	Oncogenic Ras protein that is frequently mutated in cancers. When the amino acid glycine G replaced with amino acid valine V at codon 12, it becomes permanently activated within the cell (proto-oncogene), leading to uncontrolled cell division and tumor formation.
JMJD3	Histone demethylase that promotes melanoma progression and metastasis through regulation of NF-kappa B and BMP signaling
MAPK (MAP kinase signaling pathway)	Responsible for relaying extracellular signals from cell membrane to nucleus. Dysregulation of this pathway due to activating mutations in BRAF, RAS and other genes leads to increased signaling activity leading to cell proliferation, invasion, metastasis, migration, survival, and angiogenesis.
NRAS	Member of the RAS family of GTPases (small GTPase proteins) that mediate growth factor receptor signaling and are critical for cell proliferation, survival, and differentiation. Activating mutations in NRAS proto-oncogene, particularly at codon 61, are also common in human melanoma
OIS	Oncogene-induced senescence
p16 (also p16^{INK4A})	Tumor suppressor protein that functions as a cyclin-dependent kinase inhibitor and is encoded by the CDKN2A gene. Plays a significant role in cell cycle regulation; tumor suppressor implicated in the prevention of melanoma and many other cancers. It is 1 of the genes associated with hereditary melanoma and plays a role in cell senescence.
p21^{WAF1}	Cyclin-dependent kinase inhibitor that mediates p53-dependent cell cycle arrest and likely plays a role as a tumor suppressor. This protein also inhibits apoptosis and may promote cell proliferation in some tumors.
p53	Mutation of this tumor suppressor gene is common in melanoma, more so in many other cancers. In normal cells, p53 plays a role in cell cycle arrest and DNA repair or apoptosis, and can mediate cellular senescence.
PcG	Polycomb group

PTEN (Phosphatase and tensin homolog)	Tumor suppressor gene that is frequently lost/inactivated in melanoma. The PTEN protein is a phosphatase that negatively regulates the PI3K/Akt pathway and influences cell adhesion, migration, and invasion.
PI3K-AKT pathway	Activation of this pathway is one of the most significant signaling pathways in melanoma. It plays a role in melanoma initiation and resistance to therapeutics.
PRC	Polycomb repressive complexes 1 and 2 (PRC1 and PRC2), which are protein complexes associated with chromatin condensation and transcriptional repression (epigenetic modifications) PRC1 catalyzes the ubiquitylation of histone H2A and PRC2 methylates H3K27.
RB	Tumor suppressor gene that normally arrests cells in the G1 or G1/S phase of the cell cycle by acting as a transcriptional repressor. Loss or inactivation can lead to uncontrolled cell proliferation
SAHF	Senescence-associated heterochromatic foci-Domains of condensed chromatin, or heterochromatin that form often in senescent human cells. They play a role in repressing proliferation-promoting genes and their detection can help identify senescent cells.
SA β-gal	Senescence-associated β-galactosidase activity that is detectable at pH 6.0 in cells undergoing replicative or induced senescence that us absent in proliferating cells. This is the most commonly used biomarker for senescence.
SETDB1	Histone methyltransferase that is overexpressed in melanoma and accelerates its onset in zebrafish melanoma models harboring the BRAF V600E mutation
SMAD1	Gene that encodes a protein involved in the downstream signaling pathway of BMP
SUZ12	Component of the PRC2 complex

is postulated that these nevi are a result of clonal proliferation of a melanoblast during embryogenesis.

Acquired nevi appear early in childhood, after the first year of life, and increase in number with age, peaking during the third or fourth decade of life.[4,5] Heredity and environment (ultraviolent radiation) are predisposing factors. Clinically, they are flat, superficial, and horizontally oriented lesions that are usually smaller (<6 mm in diameter) than congenital nevi. Dermatoscopically, they can have a reticular, globular, or homogeneous appearance, alone or in combination (**Fig. 1**). The distinct patterns probably correspond to different arrangements of the nested an adherent lesional melanocytes. Histologically, melanocytes in acquired nevi usually do not involve the reticular dermis or the subcutis, and the melanocytes are monomorphous and small with an oval shape.

Most melanocytic nevi either disappear or remain stable during life, with fewer than 5% undergoing detectable change when closely monitored.[6-8] However, it is estimated that 25% to 50% of cutaneous melanomas arise from melanocytic nevi as precursor lesions.[9,10] A recent meta-analysis by Lin and colleagues[11] of 13 studies involving more than 4000 cases revealed that 32% of melanomas are associated with a nevus. Risk of malignant transformation is associated with increased size of congenital nevi,[12] and risk

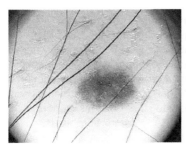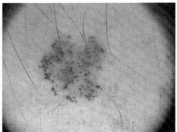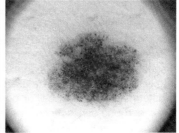

Fig. 1. Dermatoscopic patterns of acquired melanocytic nevi. (*Left*) Acquired melanocytic nevus with reticular, or net-like, pattern visible through homogeneous brown pigmentation. (*Center*) Acquired nevus with distinct globular dermatoscopic pattern. (*Right*) Acquired nevus with combined reticular and globular dermatoscopic pattern.

of cutaneous melanoma correlates with number of total and clinically dysplastic nevi.[13,14]

In contrast to their malignant counterparts, most melanocytic nevi are benign tumors that initially proliferate but remain stable or disappear during life. However, despite these differences in behavior, nevi and melanomas share somatic mutations in common. A high proportion of large and giant congenital nevi have activating mutations at codon 61 of NRAS, 1 of the 3 major isoforms of the RAS family of GTPase proteins involved in cell growth, survival, and differentiation.[15,16] Small and medium-sized congenital melanocytic nevi, as well as many acquired melanocytic nevi, contain a key mutation in the BRAF gene, resulting in substitution of glutamic acid for valine at position V600 of the protein within the kinase domain in exon 15.[17] This mutation results in constitutively active $BRAF^{V600E}$.[18] BRAF is a serine-threonine kinase that is activated by the RAS family of proteins that, when activated, triggers the MAP kinase signaling pathway (MAPK) signaling cascade. Up to 80% of benign nevi carry the $BRAF^{V600E}$ mutation.[17] Both mutations are found at high frequency in cutaneous melanomas, with the $BRAF^{V600E}$ mutation being detected in about 60% to 70% of malignant melanomas.[19] Initial correlation of somatic mutations in nevi with dermatoscopic pattern suggests that BRAF mutations may be most closely associated with globular, rather than reticular, melanocytic nevi.[20] Despite activation of the MAPK pathway, which mediates a potent proliferative signal, benign nevi lose all proliferative activity. The paradox of stable melanocytic proliferations exhibiting oncogenic mutations at high frequency led to the suggestion that melanocytic nevi represent the outcome of oncogene-induced senescence (OIS) in the skin.[21]

CELLULAR SENESCENCE

Most normal mammalian cells are unable to keep growing indefinitely. After 40 to 70 cell divisions in culture, the cell enters a state of senescence. In this state, basic metabolic processes occur but the cell neither dies nor divides, a phenomenon initially characterized by Shay and colleagues,[22] and Hayflick and Moorhead,[23] with human fibroblasts.

Senescent cells display many phenotypic changes that, individually, cannot definitively indicate senescence but can be used in combination to determine whether a cell or population of cells has undergone senescence. A major indicator of senescence is the cessation of cell division, combined with a resistance to undergo apoptosis. Another commonly accepted marker of senescent cells is the expression of β-galactosidase that is detectable at pH 6, referred to as senescence-associated β-galactosidase (SA β-gal).[24] Several other phenotypic changes are associated with senescence. Senescent cells often show a striking morphologic change: the cell flattens and may adopt a more dendritic shape.[25] Finally, a senescence-activated secretory phenotype, which is marked by an increased expression of secreted proteins, including cytokines, is activated.[26]

In addition to these cell-wide changes, several changes are also apparent on the molecular level in senescent cells. These cells show punctate condensation of their chromatin known as senescence-associated heterochromatic foci (SAHF). In addition to these chromatin changes, and, in some cases, perhaps due to these changes, there are a large number of genes that show expression changes after a cell enters senescence. Some of these genes are directly involved in the senescence process, such as the cell cycle regulators $p16^{INK4A}$ and $p21^{WAF1}$, which are induced in senescence and maintain the tumor suppressor retinoblastoma (Rb) protein in its hypophosphorylated, and active, state.[25]

Another variant of senescence, premature senescence, has been characterized. Premature senescence refers to senescence that occurs without any detectable telomere dysfunction and can be induced by various stimuli. These stimuli include environmental stress in vitro, such as suboptimal nutrient levels or oxygen tension, and oncogene activation. The phenomenon of OIS was first described as a proliferative cell cycle arrest in primary human and mouse fibroblasts, following the retroviral introduction of oncogenic $HRAS^{G12V}$. Forced expression of $HRAS^{G12V}$ in these cells results in cellular changes indistinguishable from the phenotype observed on replicative senescence, and is associated with increases in the expression of p16, p53, and p21. OIS absolutely depends on p16 and p53 in rodent cells; however, their loss is not sufficient to abrogate this effect in human cells.[27] Several mechanisms of OIS induction and escape are listed in **Table 1**.

In humans, the concept of OIS is well illustrated in the pathogenesis of melanocytic nevi. The forced expression of $BRAF^{V600E}$ in primary human melanocytes leads to a transient cellular proliferation, followed by a growth arrest and induction of p16 and SA β-gal expression as senescence markers, similar to the changes reported on expression of $HRAS^{G12V}$ in fibroblasts.[27,28] A model for the transient proliferation, followed by growth arrest and senescence, of melanocytes on oncogene activation to form a nevus is presented in **Fig. 2**.

Table 1
Mechanisms of oncogene-induced senescence induction and escape

Mechanism	Epigenetic or Signaling Consequence	Effect on Senescence
BRAF^{V600E} mutation	Constitutive activation of MAPK signaling	Senescence induction
NRAS-activating mutations	Constitutive activation of MAPK signaling	Senescence induction
p53 suppression	Abrogated DNA damage checkpoints, cell cycle changes	Suppress OIS
RB suppression	Cell cycle changes	Suppress OIS
SETDB1 overexpression	Chromatin remodeling	Suppress OIS
PI3K pathway activation	Cell cycle changes	Suppress OIS
Atg7 depletion	Increased oxidative stress	Suppress OIS
BMI-1 activation	Repression of *CDKN2A*	Suppress OIS
EZH2 activation	H3K27me3 trimethylation	Suppress OIS
NF-κβ signaling (noncanonical)	RB stabilization	Suppress OIS
CBX4	Chromatin remodeling	Suppress OIS
CBX7	Repression of *Ink4b/ARF/Ink4a*	Suppress OIS

Melanocytic nevi in vivo also express senescence markers, leading to the suggestion that OIS in human melanocytes represents a barrier to tumor progression in melanoma development[28,29] OIS has also been shown to occur in model systems. Patton and colleagues[30] showed that overexpression of BRAF^{V600E} in transgenic zebrafish led to the development of fish nevi and in mice, expression of BRAF^{V600E} in melanocytes produced nevi with biochemical evidence of senescence.[31] A concept of how acquisition of an activating *NRAS* mutation in a melanocyte precursor, or melanoblast, during embryonic development might lead to the formation of a congenital melanocytic nevus is depicted in **Fig. 3**.

MAINTENANCE AND LOSS OF SENESCENCE IN NEVI AND MELANOMA: THE ROLE OF GENETICS AND EPIGENETICS

Understanding the mechanisms underlying the breakdown of the senescence barrier, leading to

Oncogene activation and cellular senescence

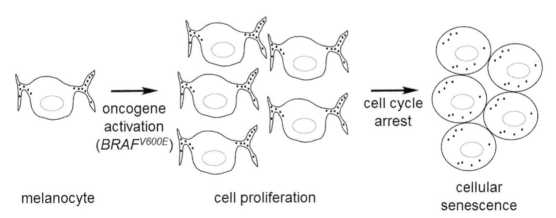

Fig. 2. Model for the development of a melanocytic nevus following activation of BRAF with acquisition of BRAF^{V600E} somatic mutation. Acquisition of the activating mutation (most likely from an unrepaired oxidative modification to guanine) results in transient melanocyte proliferation driven by MAP kinase signaling. Subsequently, a senescence response is induced and growth arrest occurs, leaving a clonal population of oncogene-harboring, melanocytic cells forming the nevus.

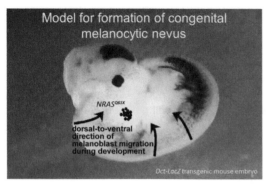

Model for formation of congenital melanocytic nevus

NRAS^Q61X

dorsal-to-ventral
direction of
melanoblast migration
during development

Dct-LacZ transgenic mouse embryo

Fig. 3. Concept for the development of large congenital melanocytic nevus following activation of NRAS following Q61 mutation in melanoblast. A mouse *Dct-lacZ* embryo[32] is shown in which individual melanoblasts are stained blue. Melanoblasts migrate from the neural tube, at the back of the embryo, across to the ventral surface. Acquisition of a somatic activating mutation at codon 61 of NRAS in a single melanoblast may lead to massive proliferation of clonal progeny before OIS results in growth arrest. (*Adapted from* Hornyak TJ, Hayes DH, Chiu LY, et al. Transcription factors in melanocyte development: distinct roles for Pax-3 and Mitf. Mech Dev 2001;101:51; with permission.)

further tumor progression, may lead to advances in maintaining or reimposing it as a therapeutic strategy. The mechanisms that these cells develop to escape OIS are largely unknown but have been explored in vitro and in vivo. **Table 1** summarizes the effects of many of the proteins and mechanisms on OIS. Studies in zebrafish have shown that OIS can be reversed in BRAF^V600E, expressing melanocytic nevus cells through experimental suppression of p53.[30] Suppression of RB function, as well as loss of the phosphatase and tensin homolog (PTEN) and overexpression of SETDB1, have similarly been shown to abrogate OIS experimentally.[33–35] Vredeveld and colleagues[36] recently demonstrated that PI3K pathway activation acts as a crucial step in melanomagenesis in vitro by terminating BRAF^V600E-induced senescence.

Essential autophagy gene autophagy-related-7 (*Atg7*) has also been shown to promote the development of melanoma in BRAF^V600E mutant *Pten-null* mice by overcoming senescence. In the same study, its loss increased oxidative stress, induced senescence, and improved the response to treatment with BRAF inhibitor dabrafenib.[37]

Melanoma therapies targeting the OIS pathway are currently under investigation. In addition to the focus on BRAF inhibitors, vemurafenib and trametinib, which are clinically efficacious,[38,39] there have also been initiatives to test these highly-selective BRAF inhibitors in combination with inhibitors of related pathways in melanomagenesis also relevant to senescence, such as PIK3CA and *Atg7*.[37,40]

Polycomb group (PcG) proteins have been implicated as mediators of cellular senescence. PcG proteins are members of distinct macromolecular complexes, the major ones being polycomb repressive complex (PRC)-1 and PRC2, which modify and interact with histones to maintain a cell's epigenetic state. The polycomb protein Bmi-1 was implicated in cellular senescence by virtue of its activity as an epigenetic repressor of the *Cdkn2a* locus, encoding the p16^Ink4a tumor suppressor, in murine cells. In human cells, overexpression of BMI-1 extended the time to replicative senescence that was associated with repression of p16 expression.[24] The enhancer of zeste homolog 2 (EZH2) is the catalytic component of the PRC2, also consisting of other key members, such as SUZ12 and embryonic ectoderm development (EED), which have not been shown to be catalytic but play structural roles. EZH2 functions as a histone methyltransferase, adding a third methyl group to the ε-amino group of lysine 27 on histone 3, generating the H3K27me3 modification that is associated with gene repression in genome-wide studies. In both replicatively and prematurely senescent cells, a reduction in the expression of EZH2 is associated with reduction in the H3K27me3 histone mark and upregulation of p16 expression at the *Cdkn2a/CDKN2A* locus.[41] A partial explanation for the reduction of the H3K27me3 mark in senescent cells was provided when it was established that, during RAS-RAF activation, the H3K27me3 demethylase JMJD3 was induced and recruited to the p16 promoter to counter PcG protein-mediated repression of *Cdkn2a* and cause the p16-dependent growth arrest characteristic of OIS.[42]

Increased expression of EZH2 is commonly observed in cancer.[43] The observation that EZH2 expression might progressively increase during melanoma progression, together with the suppression of the senescent state occurring during that process, suggested that there might be a relationship between EZH2 overexpression in melanoma cells and the suppression of the senescent state, thereby promoting melanoma development and tumorigenicity.

To confirm that EZH2 expression is associated with melanoma progression, the authors obtained specimens of benign human melanocytic nevi and metastatic melanoma tumors, and observed, on a cell-by-cell basis, a marked increase in the percentage of melanocytic cells expressing EZH2. To test the hypothesis that the induction of EZH2 expression between nevus and melanoma cells was responsible for the loss of senescence and tumor progression, we used RNA interference to suppress the expression of *EZH2* in melanoma cells with *NRAS* activating mutations. Suppression of EZH2 in these cells led to the reappearance of senescence markers, such as SA β-gal, SAHF, and H3K9me3 foci, and was also associated with other typical senescence changes, such as G1 cell cycle arrest and an increase in cell and nuclear size. Stable suppression of *EZH2* expression was also found to inhibit tumor cell colony formation in soft agar and in vivo tumor xenograft growth in immunodeficient mice.[44]

Mechanistically, the induction of senescence in melanoma cells on loss of EZH2 could not be attributed to an induction in p16 expression or activity because all of the cells tested either did not express p16 or expressed a mutated form. Instead, we detected a p53-independent induction of p21 expression in most of the EZH2-suppressed melanoma cells. This induction was found to be responsible for a significant proportion of the senescence effect (**Fig. 4**). Nevertheless, the *CDKN1A* gene encoding p21 was not found to be a direct target of EZH2, exhibiting neither significant occupancy by EZH2 nor a high concentration of H3K27me3 modifications, as is typical for direct PRC2 interaction sites, following chromatin immunoprecipitation studies. Hence the direct targets of EZH2 in melanoma genomes responsible for the repression of p21/*CDKN1A* in these cells, and the suppression of the senescent state that promotes tumor progression, remain to be described.

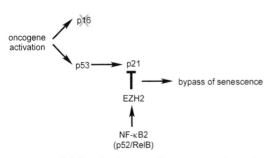

Fig. 4. Model for the bypass of senescence in melanoma cells induced by EZH2 and/or noncanonical NF-κB signaling. Senescence in melanocytes can be mediated by the tumor suppressors p16 or p53; however, p16 function is invariably inactivated in most cutaneous melanomas, whereas p53 gene sequence and function usually remains intact. EZH2 induction in melanoma cells results in senescence bypass by suppressing the expression of prosenescent p21 downstream of p53-p21 activation. EZH2 expression depends on noncanonical NF-κB signaling through the p52 and RelB subunits.

However, EZH2 expression has recently been found to be regulated by noncanonical NF-κβ signaling through stabilization of Rb via p21 and p53.[45,46] This may be an explanation for the p53-independent induction of p21 that is seen in EZH2-suppressed melanoma cells. In addition, noncanonical NF-κβ signaling was shown to prevent OIS. Continued activation of the noncanonical NF-κβ pathway in the context of EZH2 suppression would lead to an increase of p21 in an unsuccessful attempt by the cell to regulate EZH2 expression and bypass senescence. The roles of PcG proteins in melanocyte and melanoma function have been summarized.[47,48]

Additional recent studies have extended findings about the role of PcG proteins in senescence. A major role of Cbx4, a PRC1 component, is to suppress senescence of epidermal stem cells through its chromodomain and interactions with the H3 tail domain. Cbx4 expression seems to be important in these cells to fine-tune the transition of epidermal stem cells between the quiescent and active states.[49] Cbx7, another PRC1 component, mediates senescence by binding to and repressing the classic PcG protein target *Ink4b/ARF/Ink4a*. Interestingly, its ability to bind to the locus and inhibit senescence depends not only on its ability to recognize and bind H3K27me3 but also to bind *ANRIL*, a noncoding RNA transcribed from the locus that bridges the interactions between H3K27me3 and PRC1.[50] Ras-induced senescence in mouse embryonic fibroblasts is associated with dramatic changes in both H3K4me3 and H3K27me3 trimethylation that alter expression of critical components of the Bmp2-Smad1 signaling pathway, enforcing senescence through the induction of a senescence-associated secretory phenotype[51] Though each of these studies were performed using primary cells, it is likely that genome-wide chromatin immunoprecipitation studies with cancer cells will also reveal important and unrecognized polycomb-regulated genes responsible for the suppression of senescence in these cells.

SUMMARY

Melanocytic nevi most likely represent the outcome of clonal proliferation of single melanocytes that acquire highly specific, somatic mutations that escape DNA repair and cause them to proliferate to a variable extent in the skin. These particular mutations, such as mutations at BRAF[V600E] and at codon 61 in *NRAS*, likely function in a highly cell type–specific context to drive proliferation because benign tumors arising from other cell types do not feature identical mutations at high frequency. Concomitantly, expression of the oncogene induces a senescence response in the proliferating melanocytes that stops cell growth and presents a barrier to further malignant transformation. Infrequently, nevi undergo transformation to malignant melanoma. This transition is associated not only with further genetic changes, such as loss or mutation of the *CDKN2A* locus encoding the p16 tumor suppressor, but also with epigenetic changes, such as chromatin-level silencing of tumor suppressor gene expression that is also a factor in tumor progression. Polycomb proteins, including proteins comprising PRC2, have important roles in cancer development. The members of this complex have been found to be overexpressed in a variety of cancers, including melanoma. EZH2 expression increases progressively from being undetectable in normal melanocytes to low in nevi and high in melanoma, with an increase seen between primary and metastatic lesion. EZH2 depletion from melanoma cell lines has been shown to decrease proliferation, increase the percentage of cells with a senescent phenotype, and decrease the volume of tumors generated with a xenograft experiment. In addition, several mutations of EZH2 have been identified that increase the H3K27Me3 activity of the PRC2 complex in lymphoma. Growing evidence suggests that the epigenetic regulation catalyzed by PRC2 may play a role in regulating senescence. Senescence is a barrier to uncontrolled proliferation but can be bypassed. Reversing senescence bypass and rendering proliferating tumor cells dormant may, as a result, be a useful adjunct to targeted therapies and immunotherapies that are currently used for advanced melanoma, and that remain under investigation for other cutaneous malignancies.

REFERENCES

1. Argenziano G, Zalaudek I, Ferrara G, et al. Proposal of a new classification system for melanocytic naevi. Br J Dermatol 2007;157:217–27.
2. Price HN, Schaffer JV. Congenital melanocytic nevi-when to worry and how to treat: Facts and controversies. Clin Dermatol 2010;28(3):293–302.
3. Schaffer JV. Update on melanocytic nevi in children. Clin Dermatol 2015;33(3):368–86.
4. Bataille V, Grulich A, Sasieni P, et al. The association between naevi and melanoma in populations with different levels of sun exposure: a joint case-control study of melanoma in the UK and Australia. Br J Cancer 1998;77:505–10.
5. Grulich AE, Bataille V, Swerdlow AJ, et al. Naevi and pigmentary characteristics as risk factors for melanoma in a high-risk population: a case-control study in New South Wales, Australia. Int J Cancer 1996;67:485–91.
6. Haenssle HA, Krueger U, Vente C, et al. Results from an observational trial: digital epiluminescence microscopy follow-up of atypical nevi increases the sensitivity and the chance of success of conventional dermoscopy in detecting melanoma. J Invest Dermatol 2006;126:980–5.
7. Kittler H, Pehamberger H, Wolff K, et al. Follow-up of melanocytic skin lesions with digital epiluminescence microscopy: patterns of modifications observed in early melanoma, atypical nevi, and common nevi. J Am Acad Dermatol 2000;43:467–76.
8. Robinson JK, Nickoloff BJ. Digital epiluminescence microscopy monitoring of high-risk patients. Arch Dermatol 2004;140:49–56.
9. Bevona C, Goggins W, Quinn T, et al. Cutaneous melanomas associated with nevi. Arch Dermatol 2003;139:1620–4 [discussion: 1624].
10. Sagebiel RW. Melanocytic nevi in histologic association with primary cutaneous melanoma of superficial spreading and nodular types: effect of tumor thickness. J Invest Dermatol 1993;100:322S–5S.
11. Lin WM, Luo S, Muzikansky A, et al. Outcome of patients with de novo versus nevus-associated melanoma. J Am Acad Dermatol 2015;72(1):54–8.
12. Egan CL, Oliveria SA, Elenitsas R, et al. Cutaneous melanoma risk and phenotypic changes in large congenital nevi: a follow-up study of 46 patients. J Am Acad Dermatol 1998;39:923–32.
13. Tucker MA, Halpern A, Holly EA, et al. Clinically recognized dysplastic nevi. A central risk factor for cutaneous melanoma. JAMA 1997;277:1439–44.
14. Newton-Bishop JA, Chang YM, Iles MM, et al. Melanocytic nevi, nevus genes, and melanoma risk in a large case-control study in the United Kingdom. Cancer Epidemiol Biomarkers Prev 2010;19:2043–54.
15. Bauer J, Curtin JA, Pinkel D, et al. Congenital melanocytic nevi frequently harbor NRAS mutations but no BRAF mutations. J Invest Dermatol 2006;127:179–82.
16. Roh MR, Eliades P, Gupta S, et al. Genetics of melanocytic nevi. Pigment Cell Melanoma Res 2015;28:661–72.
17. Pollock PM, Harper UL, Hansen KS, et al. High frequency of BRAF mutations in nevi. Nat Genet 2003;33:19–20.
18. Wellbrock C, Ogilvie L, Hedley D, et al. V599EB-RAF is an oncogene in melanocytes. Cancer Res 2004;64:2338–42.
19. Curtin JA, Fridlyand J, Kageshita T, et al. Distinct sets of genetic alterations in melanoma. N Engl J Med 2005;353:2135–47.
20. Marchetti MA, Kiuru MH, Busam KJ, et al. Melanocytic naevi with globular and reticular dermoscopic patterns display distinct BRAF V600E expression profiles and histopathological patterns. Br J Dermatol 2014;171:1060–5.

21. Bennett DC. Human melanocyte senescence and melanoma susceptibility genes. Oncogene 2003; 22:3063–9.

22. Shay JW, Wright WE. Hayflick, his limit, and cellular ageing. Nat Rev Mol Cell Biol 2000;1:72–6.

23. Hayflick L, Moorhead PS. The serial cultivation of human diploid cell strains. Exp Cell Res 1961;25: 585–621.

24. Dimri GP, Lee X, Basile G, et al. A biomarker that identifies senescent human cells in culture and in aging skin in vivo. Proc Natl Acad Sci U S A 1995; 92(20):9363–7.

25. Campisi J, D'adda Di Fagagna F. Cellular senescence: when bad things happen to good cells. Nat Rev Mol Cell Biol 2007;8:729–40.

26. Coppe JP, Patil CK, Rodier F, et al. Senescence-associated secretory phenotypes reveal cell-nonautonomous functions of oncogenic RAS and the p53 tumor suppressor. PLoS Biol 2008;6:2853–68.

27. Serrano M, Lin AW, Mccurrach ME, et al. Oncogenic ras provokes premature cell senescence associated with accumulation of p53 and p16INK4a. Cell 1997; 88:593–602.

28. Michaloglou C, Vredeveld LC, Soengas MS, et al. BRAFE600-associated senescence-like cell cycle arrest of human naevi. Nature 2005;436:720–4.

29. Gray-Schopfer VC, Cheong SC, Chong H, et al. Cellular senescence in naevi and immortalisation in melanoma: a role for p16? Br J Cancer 2006;95:496–505.

30. Patton EE, Widlund HR, Kutok JL, et al. BRAF mutations are sufficient to promote nevi formation and cooperate with p53 in the genesis of melanoma. Curr Biol 2005;15:249–54.

31. Goel VK, Ibrahim N, Jiang G, et al. Melanocytic nevus-like hyperplasia and melanoma in transgenic BRAFV600E mice. Oncogene 2009;28:2289–98.

32. Hornyak TJ, Hayes DH, Chiu LY, et al. Transcription factors in melanocyte development: distinct roles for Pax-3 and Mitf. Mech Dev 2001;101:47–59.

33. Ceol CJ, Houvras Y, Jane-Valbuena J, et al. The histone methyltransferase SETDB1 is recurrently amplified in melanoma and accelerates its onset. Nature 2011;471:513–7.

34. Dankort D, Curley DP, Cartlidge RA, et al. Braf(V600E) cooperates with Pten loss to induce metastatic melanoma. Nat Genet 2009;41:544–52.

35. Sage J, Mulligan GJ, Attardi LD, et al. Targeted disruption of the three Rb-related genes leads to loss of G(1) control and immortalization. Genes Dev 2000;14:3037–50.

36. Vredeveld LC, Possik PA, Smit MA, et al. Abrogation of BRAFV600E-induced senescence by PI3K pathway activation contributes to melanomagenesis. Genes Dev 2012;26:1055–69.

37. Xie X, Koh JY, Price S, et al. Atg7 overcomes senescence and promotes growth of BrafV600E-driven melanoma. Cancer Discov 2015;5:410–23.

38. Chapman PB, Hauschild A, Robert C, et al. Improved survival with vemurafenib in melanoma with BRAF V600E mutation. N Engl J Med 2011; 364:2507–16.

39. Flaherty KT, Infante JR, Daud A, et al. Combined BRAF and MEK inhibition in melanoma with BRAF V600 mutations. N Engl J Med 2012;367:1694–703.

40. Liu C, Peng W, Xu C, et al. BRAF inhibition increases tumor infiltration by T cells and enhances the anti-tumor activity of adoptive immunotherapy in mice. Clin Cancer Res 2013;19:393–403.

41. Bracken AP, Kleine-Kohlbrecher D, Dietrich N, et al. The polycomb group proteins bind throughout the INK4A-ARF locus and are disassociated in senescent cells. Genes Dev 2007;21:525–30.

42. Agger K, Cloos PA, Rudkjaer L, et al. The H3K27me3 demethylase JMJD3 contributes to the activation of the INK4A-ARF locus in response to oncogene- and stress-induced senescence. Genes Dev 2009;23:1171–6.

43. Kleer CG, Cao Q, Varambally S, et al. EZH2 is a marker of aggressive breast cancer and promotes neoplastic transformation of breast epithelial cells. Proc Natl Acad Sci U S A 2003;100:11606–11.

44. Fan T, Jiang S, Chung N, et al. EZH2-dependent suppression of a cellular senescence phenotype in melanoma cells by inhibition of p21/CDKN1A expression. Mol Cancer Res 2011;9:418–29.

45. Iannetti A, Ledoux AC, Tudhope SJ, et al. Regulation of p53 and Rb links the alternative NF-kappaB pathway to EZH2 expression and cell senescence. PLoS Genet 2014;10:e1004642.

46. De Donatis GM, Pape EL, Pierron A, et al. NF-kB2 induces senescence bypass in melanoma via a direct transcriptional activation of EZH2. Oncogene 2015; 35(21):2735–45.

47. Tiffen J, Gallagher SJ, Hersey P. EZH2: an emerging role in melanoma biology and strategies for targeted therapy. Pigment Cell Melanoma Res 2015;28:21–30.

48. Huang JM, Hornyak TJ. Polycomb group proteins–epigenetic repressors with emerging roles in melanocytes and melanoma. Pigment Cell Melanoma Res 2015;28:330–9.

49. Luis NM, Morey L, Mejetta S, et al. Regulation of human epidermal stem cell proliferation and senescence requires polycomb- dependent and -independent functions of Cbx4. Cell Stem Cell 2011;9:233–46.

50. Yap KL, Li S, Munoz-Cabello AM, et al. Molecular interplay of the noncoding RNA ANRIL and methylated histone H3 lysine 27 by polycomb CBX7 in transcriptional silencing of INK4a. Mol Cell 2010;38:662–74.

51. Kaneda A, Fujita T, Anai M, et al. Activation of Bmp2-Smad1 signal and its regulation by coordinated alteration of H3K27 trimethylation in Ras-induced senescence. PLoS Genet 2011;7:e1002359.

Distinct Fibroblasts in the Papillary and Reticular Dermis: Implications for Wound Healing

David T. Woodley, MD

KEYWORDS

- Papillary dermis • Reticular dermis • Fibroblasts • Markers for fibroblast lineages
- Reparative wound healing • Regenerative wound healing • Scarring

KEY POINTS

- Human skin wounds heal largely by reparative wound healing rather than regenerative wound healing.
- Human skin wounds heal with scarring and without pilosebaceous units or other appendages.
- Dermal fibroblasts come from 2 distinct lineages of cells, one lineage populates the papillary dermis and the other lineage populates the reticular dermis, that have distinct cell markers and, more importantly, distinct functional abilities.
- Human skin wound healing largely involves the dermal fibroblast lineage from the reticular dermis and not the papillary dermis.
- If scientists could find a way to stimulate the dermal fibroblast lineages from the papillary dermis in early wound healing, perhaps human skin wounds could heal without scarring and with skin appendages.

INTRODUCTION

The skin is visible and readily accessible to the patient and physicians. Since the beginning of humanity, humans have manipulated their skin for medical reasons and cosmetic purposes. It has long been recognized that when surgical intervention of the skin occurs and wounding ensues at a certain depth that the skin heals with an expected scar that lacks hair and other skin appendages. Even naturally occurring diseases appear to respect a similar biological rule. The autoimmune bullous disease, pemphigus vulgaris, has an intra-epidermal blister that tends to heal without scarring. In contrast, another bullous disease, dystrophic epidermolysis bullosa (DEB), features a deeper blister cleavage plane beneath the epidermal-dermal junction (specifically below the lamina densa area of the basement membrane zone), and these blisters, unlike pemphigus blister, uniformly heal with exuberant scarring. When we are talking literally about a few nanometers difference of skin depth in this direction or that direction, why is the advent of scarring or no scarring so incredibly predictable? It appears to be due to a unique lineage of fibroblasts that inhabit the papillary dermis.

The average dermatologist does between 750 and 1000 skin biopsies per year. Many of these biopsies are taken with a punch biopsy tool that ranges in size from 2 mm to 15 mm in diameter. The usual "punch biopsy" for diagnosis is usually 2 to 4 mm in size. This type of biopsy goes down through the epidermis and dermis into the subcutaneous fat, hypodermis. **Fig. 1** shows the

Disclosure: This work was partially funded by a VA Merit Review Grant.
Department of Dermatology, The Keck School of Medicine, University of Southern California, USC/Norris Cancer Center, Topping Tower 3405, 1441 Eastlake Avenue, Los Angeles, CA 90033, USA
E-mail address: david.woodley@med.usc.edu

Dermatol Clin 35 (2017) 95–100
http://dx.doi.org/10.1016/j.det.2016.07.004

histology of such a biopsy specimen. The outer epidermal layer consists largely of epidermal keratinocytes. Interspersed within the epidermis, there are other nonkeratinocyte cells with special functions. Interspersed within the basal layer of keratinocytes there are dendritic melanocytes that make melanin and eumelanin that imparts color to the skin. Within the midepidermis there are other dendritic cells called Langerhans cells that sense invading antigens in the skin and are outposts for mounting an immune response. They are professional antigen-presenting cells and process external antigens and present them to the immune system. Last, in the epidermis there are Merkel cells, which are in association with unmyelinated free nerve endings and function to impart tactile sensory perception and light touch discrimination to the skin. The epidermis is relatively thin (0.04 mm on the eyelids), 1.6 mm, depending on the location (1.6 mm on the palms of a young adult). The average thickness of the epidermis is 0.1 mm.[1] Nevertheless, regardless of what location of the body is examined, the dermis overall is 15 to 40 times thicker than the epidermis, depending on the anatomic site.[1] Although the dermis may contain variable numbers of mast cells, lymphocytes, dendritic cells, and vascular endothelial cells, the main "work horse" cell for the dermis is the dermal fibroblast, spindle-shaped mesenchymal cells, which make all of the dermal components and also have the machinery to modulate and turn over dermal extracellular matrix components (ECMs). During early wound healing, the skin needs to reconstitute itself. The rent in the skin is initially filled with a fibrin clot containing fibrin, fibrinogen, fibronectin, and fragments of collagen. To resurface the wound and make an underlying vascular neodermis, 3 processes must occur: reepithelialization, fibroplasia, and neovascularization. These 3 processes require the migration of 3 critical skin cells. Keratinocytes at the cut edges of the wound need to reprogram themselves and, rather than differentiate into a stratified squamous epithelium and Stratum corneum, must become motile cells and laterally migrate across the wound bed, the process of "reepithelialization." The clot in the wound is the initial wound bed and must transform into a neodermis. This requires the migration of periwound fibroblasts into the clot to begin laying down new collagen and other ECMs of the neodermis, the process of "fibroplasia." The neodermis must reestablish its blood supply and this requires the ingress of periwound microvascular endothelial cells into the clot to establish new vascular tubes in the neodermis.[2] To repair a skin wound, these 3 cells must all migrate and this migration requires an orchestration that likely involves epidermal-mesenchymal cell interactions.

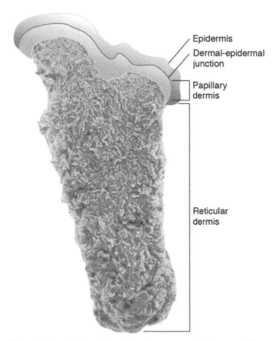

Epidermis
Dermal-epidermal junction
Papillary dermis
Reticular dermis

Fig. 1. Vertical section of a 4-mm punch biopsy taken from the shoulder. Note that the epidermis (*pseudo-colored light gray*) and papillary dermis (*pseudo-colored green*) comprise a small percentage of the total thickness of the skin. The coarsely fibered reticular dermis (*pseudo-colored yellow*) is composed mainly of type I collagen and contributes most the total thickness of the skin. Nevertheless, even a disease process causing intraepidermal blisters, such as pemphigus vulgaris, can be a life-threatening disease despite a fully intact dermis.

PAPILLARY DERMIS AND RETICULAR DERMIS

Dermatopathologists have long noted that the dermis has 2 main compartments: the papillary dermis and the reticular dermis. In contrast with the very cellular avascular epidermis, the dermis appears to be composed mainly of noncellular connective tissue composed of collagen fibers, elastic fibers, and ground substance.[1] The papillary dermis resides just beneath the epidermis and appears to have a loosely arranged fine meshwork of connective tissue fibers.[3] The papillary dermis, as shown in **Fig. 1**, is a relatively thin zone just beneath the dermal-epidermal junction. In contrast, the reticular dermis is much thicker and has coarser, more compacted connective tissue fibers that run in various directions, but in a general plane parallel with the skin surface.[3] In addition, in the papillary dermis there appear to be more fibroblasts than in the reticular dermis, and these papillary fibroblasts appear more active.

Human dermal fibroblasts are capable of synthesizing and depositing into the extracellular space all of the component of the dermis. The components of the dermis include collagens, glycoproteins, proteoglycans (also called "ground substance" and "mucopolysaccharides"), and elastic fibers. The main collagen in the dermis is type I collagen and approximately 70% of the dry weight of the dermis is collagen. In unwounded, adult skin, the ratio of collagen I to collagen III is roughly 4 to 1, whereas collagen III is roughly 1:1 in neonatal skin. Type III collagen also is temporarily increased when skin is wounded and a neodermis is formed. In newly healed human skin, the ratio of collagen I and III is roughly 1:1, similar to neonatal skin. Elastic fibers are readily seen in the reticular dermis with special stains, but are not fully formed in the papillary dermis. In the reticular dermis, elastic fibers are composed of amorphous elastin surrounding microfibrils within the center of elastic fibers. Nevertheless, as the elastic fibers in the reticular dermis approach the upper limits of this compartment and interdigitate into the papillary dermis, they lose their elastin component at the interface of the papillary and reticular dermis. The microfibrils, however, continue into the interface of the papillary and reticular dermis and exist in the papillary dermis as "naked" microfibrils. They organize themselves horizontally with the surface of the skin as elaunin fibers and then vertically into the papillary dermis as oxytalan fibers. Therefore, another observation that distinguishes the papillary dermis from the reticular dermis is the presence of naked microfibrils configured as elaunin fibers and oxytalan fibers.

CLINICAL IMPORTANCE OF THE PAPILLARY DERMIS AND RETICULAR DERMIS

Little was known about why human skin had a papillary dermis and a reticular dermis or what accounted for the differences in these 2 areas of the dermis. Clinicians, however, realized that if they perturbed the skin by dermabrasion or by CO_2 laser resurfacing, and if they destroyed the skin deeper than the papillary dermis and went into the reticular dermis, that this could risk permanent scarring. In the pilosebaceous units traversing the skin and going through the epidermis and dermis, the sebaceous gland was found to enter into the pilosebaceous unit right at the interface between the papillary dermis and reticular dermis. To improve rhytids or acne scars, skin surgeons learned to destroy the surface skin down to the interface between the papillary and reticular dermis where a distinct yellowish color could be observed when the sebaceous glands were revealed and not go deeper. Going deeper into the reticular dermis could result in a permanent fibrotic process such that the skin is firm and lacks hair follicles, sebaceous glands, and eccrine glands similar to the healed skin of a full-thickness burn wound.

WHY WE HAVE A PAPILLARY AND RETICULAR DERMIS

Very recently, clues as to what accounts for the differences in the papillary dermis and reticular dermis have been discovered. It appears from the recent work of Ryan R. Driskell and coworkers[4] that the 2 layers of the dermis are formed by different lineages of dermal fibroblasts. Lineage 1 forms the papillary dermis and the dermal papillae that regulate the growth of hair follicles and arrector pili muscles. Lineage 1 fibroblasts are required for hair growth. In contrast, Lineage 2 fibroblasts form the reticular dermis and the underlying adipose layer called "the hypodermis." This discovery was made by probing mouse skin throughout development into postnatal life with antibodies to known "fibroblast markers". A total of 19 antibodies to previously published fibroblast markers were used. In mice, these 2 lineages of fibroblasts could readily be discerned by studying fibroblasts from their skin at postnatal day 2. If these cells were probed with antibodies to fibroblast markers, it was found that all of the cells in the dermis of mice expressed certain fibroblast markers, such as the platelet-derived growth factor receptor alpha (PDGFRα) throughout all stages of development.[4] In contrast, however, the fibroblasts in the papillary dermis alone stained positively for cluster

Table 1
Selected fibroblast marks staining the papillary dermis and reticular dermis in late gestation/ postnatal skin

Cell Marker	Papillary Dermis	Reticular Dermis
PDGFR alpha	Positive	Positive
CD34	Positive	Positive
BLIMP 1	Positive	Negative
CD26	Positive	Negative
Lrig1	Positive	Negative
Sca1	Negative	Positive
DLK1	Negative	Positive

Abbreviations: BLIMP, B-lymphocyte-induced maturation protein; CD, cluster differentiation; DLK1, Delta-like homologue 1; Lrig1, leucine-rich repeats and immunoglobulin like domains protein 1; PDGFR alpha, platelet-derived growth factor receptor alpha; Sca1, stem cells antigen 1.

differentiation 26 (CD26, also known as DPP4) and B-lymphocyte-induced maturation protein (BLIMP), but had negative staining for Stem Cells Antigen 1 (Sca1, also known as Ly6a). In contrast, the reticular dermal fibroblasts exhibited negative staining with antibodies to CD26 and BLIMP and positive staining for Sca1. Another marker, delta-like homologue 1 (DLK1) exhibited positive staining in the reticular dermis and negative staining in the papillary dermis. Therefore, the fibroblasts in these 2 compartments all had like staining with antibodies to PDGFRα and were defined as fibroblasts, but had opposite staining characteristics with other antibodies to fibroblast markers. This defined 2 distinct pools of dermal fibroblasts. This differential staining of papillary dermal

fibroblasts and reticular dermal fibroblasts is outlined in **Table 1**. In addition to these findings in the development of mouse skin, similar findings were found in human skin.

Having defined in whole skin papillary dermal fibroblasts and reticular dermal fibroblasts by immunostaining, these investigators next isolated fibroblasts from skin and subjected them to cell sorting by using the same antibody markers. They then had suspensions of these 2 distinct fibroblast populations. These sorted cells were then used in a well-described experimental model. In this murine model, a silicone bubble–like chamber is sewn onto the panniculus carnosus of the back of immunocompromised mice. Suspensions of keratinocytes can be mixed with suspensions of dermal fibroblast and injected into the silicone chamber. Somewhat miraculously, this mixed cell suspension "sorts" itself into a tissue that resembles skin with an epidermal layer and dermal layer (**Fig. 2**). These 2 layers are separated at the dermal-epidermal junction by basement membrane components, such as type VII collagen and anchoring fibrils.[5] Using this model, Driskell and coworkers[4] injected into the silicon chambers CD26+, BLIMP+ Sca1– cells (ie, a suspension of papillary dermal cells) and DLK1+ Sca1– cells (ie, a suspension of reticular dermal cells). When these cells sorted themselves into a skinlike tissue within the chamber, the CD26+, BLIMP+, Sca1– cells formed the papillary dermis, dermal papillae cells that regular hair development and growth and arrector pili muscle cells, whereas the other fibroblast suspension cells formed the reticular dermis and aspects of the adipose hypodermis. Remarkably, these cell lineages could be removed from whole skin, isolated into pure suspensions of cells, and they then sorted themselves in the transplanted silicon chambers grafted onto mice and

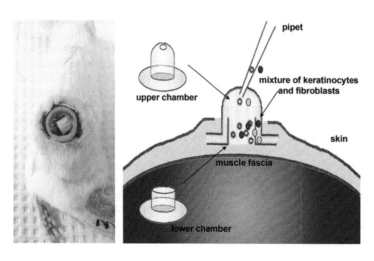

Fig. 2. Cell-sorted skin equivalent onto SCID mice. Mouse model of human skin cell suspensions sorting themselves into a human skinlike tissue with an epidermal layer, basement membrane, and dermis. A silicon chamber is sewn over the *panniculus carnosus* of the mouse. The chamber is filled with culture medium and then suspensions of human keratinocytes and human fibroblasts are injected into the chamber. Within a week, the injected keratinocytes have formed an epidermal layer and the injected fibroblasts have formed a neodermis.

reconstituted a skinlike tissue with the proper papillary dermal and reticular dermal compartments reestablished in the skin tissue.

By mixing and matching these distinct dermal fibroblast lineages in this cell-sorting skin model, it was also shown that the CD26+, BLIMP+, Sca1− cells were permissive and required for hair follicle development. The CD26−, BLIMP−, DLK1+ fibroblasts could make only the reticular dermis and parts of the hypodermis. Taken together, this study showed in an in vitro/in vivo model of cell sorting that these 2 populations or lineages of dermal fibroblasts are programmed to form either the papillary dermis with hair follicles and arrector pili muscles or a reticular dermis/hypodermis.

REPARATIVE WOUND HEALING VERSUS REGENERATIVE WOUND HEALING

Human skin wounds heal with scarring and without the reformation of skin appendages (hair follicles, eccrine glands, sebaceous glands). This is quite evident in badly burned individuals who have scarred, shiny, dry, hairless skin after their burns heal. This type of healing is called "reparative wound healing." This type of healing in mammals is quite different from lower animals, such as the newt. One can cut an entire limb from the newt and the newt will regrow an entirely new functional limb.[6] This is called "regenerative wound healing." The Holy Grail in human wound healing is to figure out how humans can heal their wounds by "regenerative wound healing" without scarring and with a full complement of functional skin appendages. Is human skin capable of "regenerative wound healing" like the newt and other amphibians? The answer is maybe. It has been shown that the human fetus is capable of repairing skin wounds made within the first trimester of gestation without scar formation.[7,8] The mechanism of how this happens is not clear, but both newt limb regeneration and scarless fetal skin healing require neural stimulation for tissue regeneration to occur.[8] Further, it appears that matrix metalloproteinases that release cells from matrix so they can continue their migratory mode are required for normal newt limb regeneration,[9] just as they are required for human skin cells to migrate, the necessary requirement for reepithelialization, fibroplasia, and neovascularization.[2]

There is an old adage that "skin wound healing is a recapitulation of gestation." Therefore, Driskell and colleagues[4] wished to determine what happens when a skin wound is made and how do the 2 lineages of fibroblasts contribute to a healed skin wound. They made full-thickness wounds on the backs of adult mice and found that the healed neodermis of healing skin wound was contributed almost exclusively by the reticular dermis lineage of fibroblasts that are incapable of making hair follicles and that reconstitute a collagen-rich extracellular matrix reminiscent of a scar. The investigators concluded that the "first wave" of dermal regeneration in skin wounds comes from those fibroblasts that are programmed and destined to be reticular dermal and hypodermal fibroblasts: a lineage that is not programmed to make hair follicles or other skin appendages.

This work gives us clues as to how scientists could perhaps achieve "regenerative healing" of skin wounds. It appears that there needs to be in the brew of wound healing and the formation of a neodermis, a distinct set of fibroblasts programmed to develop the papillary dermal dermis, a loose meshwork of fine fibers that are permissive to hair follicle formation. Mice are more plastic than human beings. In mice, it appears that when the epidermal keratinocytes begin to migrate laterally and reepithelialize a wound, these reepithelializing cells induce the papillary dermis lineage of fibroblasts in the skin. Using a conditional mouse line in which they could continuously stimulate WNT signaling and epidermal beta catenin expression in reepithelializing wounds of mice, Driskell and coworkers[4] were able to promote the formation of a papillary dermis and hair follicles in the healing wounds. Newts and salamanders have an unusual degree of cellular plasticity near the site of injury, allowing them to regenerate their limbs. The first step in this process is that epithelial cells at the wound site convert into highly migratory cells that cover the wound within a day, somewhat analogous to reepithelialization of human skin by laterally migrating human keratinocytes resurfacing the wound bed/neodermis. In the newt, after this epithelial cell covering of the limb wound, the internal mesenchymal limb cells begin to de-differentiate into a mass of progenitor cells.[9] This might be analogous to the processes in human skin of fibroplasia and neovascularization leading to granulation tissue in the wound and the initiation of a neodermis. Migrating human keratinocytes orchestrate reepithelialization by secreting heat shock protein 90 alpha (hsp90 α) a molecule that under physiologic conditions is an intracellular chaperone molecule. Under the stress of a skin wound and sudden hypoxia, the migrating keratinocytes secrete hsp90 α into the wound bed where it stimulates the keratinocytes to migrate as an autocrine "motogen" and stimulates the periwound fibroblasts and microvascular endothelial cells to migrate as a paracrine "motogen."[2] In the newt, the newly formed migrating epithelial cells are required for the growth and regeneration of the newt's limb.[9,10] The observation of Driskell and co-workers[4] that the migrating keratinocytes via Wnt signaling and sustained expression of beta catenin promote the papillary dermis lineage of fibroblasts required for appendage formation may have a parallel in human skin to the healing of a newt limb in that the migrating keratinocytes are orchestrating the mesenchymal responses. This is another example of how the epidermis and dermis influence each other. These observations may provide clues of how we might use this kind of information for devising wound-healing therapies that lead to less skin scarring and regeneration of skin appendages. It feels that the future key to regenerative wound healing is right there before our eyes, and yet we cannot yet quite see it.

REFERENCES

1. Ackerman AB. Histologic diagnosis of inflammatory skin diseases: an algorithmic method based on pattern analysis. In: Embryologic, histologic and anatomic aspects. 2nd edition. Baltimore (MD): Williams and Wilkins; 1997. p. 4. Chapter 1.

2. Woodley DT, Li W, Wysong A, et al. Keratinocyte migration and a hypothetical new role for extracellular heat shock protein alpha in orchestrating skin wound healing. Adv Wound Care 2015;4:203–12.

3. Okun MR, Edelstein LM, Fisher BK. Gross and microscopic pathology of the skin. In: Normal histology of the skin. 2nd edition. Canton (MA): Dermatopathology Foundation Press; 1988. p. 32. Chapter 2.

4. Driskell RR, Lichtenberger BM, Host E, et al. Distinct fibroblast lineages determine dermal architecture in skin development and repair. Nature 2013;504:227–81.

5. Chen M, Keene DR, Chan LS, et al. Restoration of type VII collagen expression and function in dystrophic epidermolysis bullosa. Nat Genet 2002;32: 670–5.

6. Donaldson DJ, Mahan JT, Smith GN Jr. Newt epidermal cell migration in vitro and in vivo appears to involve Arg-Gly-Asp-Ser receptors. J Cell Sci 1987;87:525–34.

7. Longaker MT, Adzick NS. The biology of fetal wound healing: a review. Plast Reconstr Surg 1991;87:788–90.

8. Stelnicki EJ, Doolabh V, Lee S, et al. Nerve dependency in scarless fetal wound healing. Plast Reconstr Surg 2000;105(1):140–7.

9. Vinarsky V, Atkinson DL, Stevenson TJ, et al. Normal newt limb regeneration requires matrix metalloproteinase function. Dev Biol 2005;279:86–98.

10. Mescher AL. Effects on adult newt limb regeneration of partial and complete skin flaps over the amputation surface. J Exp Zool 1976;195:117–28.

Index

Dermatol Clin 35 (2017) 101–105
http://dx.doi.org/10.1016/S0733-8635(16)30124-3
0733-8635/17

Moving?

Make sure your subscription moves with you!

To notify us of your new address, find your **Clinics Account Number** (located on your mailing label above your name), and contact customer service at:

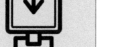

Email: journalscustomerservice-usa@elsevier.com

800-654-2452 (subscribers in the U.S. & Canada)
314-447-8871 (subscribers outside of the U.S. & Canada)

Fax number: 314-447-8029

Elsevier Health Sciences Division
Subscription Customer Service
3251 Riverport Lane
Maryland Heights, MO 63043

*To ensure uninterrupted delivery of your subscription, please notify us at least 4 weeks in advance of move.

Printed and bound by CPI Group (UK) Ltd, Croydon, CR0 4YY

03/10/2024

01040383-0007